I Will Go On

I Will Go On

Living with a Movement Disorder

Dr. Daniel Brooks

Dedication and Acknowledgement

This book is dedicated with all my love to my wife, Karrie, who has stood hand in hand with me through all of life's joys and greatest challenges. Where would I be without you? Secondly, I dedicate this book to our grown children: Stephen, Mark, Daniel, and his wife, Jenny. Your bravery, sensitivity and desire to assist me in any way possible, has sustained me. You are my pride and inspiration.

Hugs to Jamie—our faithful Labrador retriever who was by my side as I worked on my laptop.

Special Thanks to my parents, Ronald and Marguerite, my brothers, Matthew and Casey, and my sister, Teri, who have faced this difficulty with courage and understanding.

Special appreciation to those who contributed their stories, poems and emails to this book. You have motivated me to complete this task.

∽

A word of thanks to the following: Magnolia Presbyterian Church, Riverside; all of our friends in our Parkinson's support groups; friends and extended family members; online support group friends; my fellow Parkinson's and Parkinson's Plus Syndromes on-line bloggers.

I would like to thank Karrie Brooks for all of her time and skill in reading and re-reading the final transcript for errors. "Heart You."

∽

Love and gratitude to all. — Dan

Visit the We Will Go On blog at: http://WeWillGoOn.blogspot.com/ (Formerly: PD Plus Me blog)

I Will Go On
Living with a Movement Disorder

Table of Contents

Preface ~ I Will Go On

A Note from the Author

When I realized that an Abnormal Involuntary Movement Disorder was changing the direction of my life, I determined that I would write a book about how I dealt with and faced the challenges this brought, head on. I wanted to begin making an impact immediately, so I started writing a blog site on the internet entitled, "PD Plus Me." The writings of this blog were edited and revised to become a major portion of the body of this work.

As a patient, and a former educational leader, I was very motivated to learn as much as I could, so I read every book and webpage that I found relevant. I have listed many of those sources for you, with the internet sites shown at the conclusion of Chapter Three, and the book references compiled after the conclusion of the last chapter. It is my hope that you might find these references useful, as I did.

Introduction

This book will focus on the nature of Parkinson's-like conditions and the effects of these syndromes on the lives of those who suffer with them. Parkinson's Plus affects the brain in a number of areas, in addition to those that are harmed in Parkinson's Disease. Progressive Supranuclear Palsy and Multiple Systems Atrophy are among the better known conditions, but the general public knows little of these diseases. Dudley Moore died from complications of PSP, while Johnny Cash succumbed to Multiple Systems Atrophy.

Often Parkinson's Plus is referred to as Parkinson's Disease, but there are major differences in the rate of progression and the aggressiveness of the degenerative process that takes place in the brain. As the brain atrophies, the symptoms will also worsen and affect speech, swallowing, balance, walking, tremors, eye movements, bodily functions, facial expression, and cause stiffness. This list does not encompass all of the symptoms caused by Parkinson's Plus, as will be explained in more detail as you read further in this book. Cognition, meaning the thinking processes, is affected, and cognitive issues are among the least noticed, but most severe aspects of Parkinson's Plus. Each patient's case is uniquely different and no two individuals have the same list of medical issues or challenges that result from these neurological conditions.

Purpose

Why another book focusing on Parkinson's Disease or Parkinson's-like conditions you ask? There are a number of good
books on the market which discuss in detail Parkinson's Disease,
defining it and exploring a variety of treatments from medication, to herbal remedies and holistic processes that add hope to
an otherwise very disappointing, if not eventually, debilitating
struggle. No, I don't intend to provide another guide in an effort
to match some of the great editions already in print such as:
The First Year: Parkinson's Disease by Jackie Hunt Christensen,
What your Doctor May Not Tell You About Parkinson's Disease
written by Jill Marjama-Lyons, M.D. and Mary J. Shomon, and finally, 100 Questions and Answers about Parkinson's Disease by
one of the foremost experts on the condition, Abraham Lieberman, M.D. I have great respect for these excellent publications,
and it is apparent to me that books such as these have provided
a good body of knowledge about the specifics of Parkinson's
Disease and the resulting physical and emotional dilemmas it
brings in its path. Each one touches briefly, but succinctly, on
Parkinson's Plus as a similar condition that is sometimes confused with Parkinson's Disease.

However, books and materials on Parkinson's Plus are a different story all together. Medical references and professional pe-
riodicals are plentiful on the subject of Parkinson's Plus diseases, but a book for the patient and family, written by an actual

Parkinson's Plus patient is a rare find. This is the gap I have chosen to fill as my mission for the book you are now holding.

I do intend to refer to these and other books I have listed two paragraphs above, and I will provide a bibliography of materials such as these that I have depended on to get through what has been, literally, my first three years in facing Parkinsonism and the physical and mental challenges the associated symptoms and conditions have brought into my life. In writing this book I have sought to address some of the issues that haven't been given enough attention, from my perspective.

This book is for you, if you, or someone you care deeply about, has recently been diagnosed with a movement disorder with an emphasis on Parkinsonism. Parkinsonism is a broad term that refers to all conditions from idiopathic Parkinson's Disease as well as the Parkinson's Plus Syndromes. My specific diagnosis is Parkinson's Plus, and after learning that I was facing this neuro-degenerative disease, I began to write a good portion of what is in this book as a website blog, known as "PD Plus Me." The blog was so successful in attracting readers and supporters, that I soon realized a book on this subject would be a needed resource for all those I am meeting in this on-line environment, as well as community support groups for Parkinsonism sufferers in which my wife and I are involved. You will read of how frustrating it is to get diagnosed and the pitfalls of working through the medical insurance system in order to get to an accurate diagnosis and proper treatment. We will tackle the tough questions of how this affects:

- Your confidence in your future well-being

- Explaining the disease you have to your spouse, children, siblings and parents

- Adjusting your career expectations, especially for those facing an early onset, or midlife onset, of this serious illness

- Finding a balance between your treatment, need for rest and remaining focused on your life goals

- Seeking help for the emotional issues that having this serious condition brings

- Why do your friends and relatives comments, such as, "You don't look that bad to me," cause you to feel hurt or anger?

- Dealing with the loss of driving, walking and other resulting changes stemming from disabling issues associated with Parkinson's

- Making the most of every day and recognizing that your life will go on with some adjustments.

This book has been written in a biographical style, in that I have shared my own personal experiences, spiritual insights and emotional reactions in and amongst the disease information, suggestions and recommendations I have provided. In the coming chapters, you will learn how the various Parkinson's Plus diseases are defined and what physical and cognitive functions are affected. I will include writings about my personal journey for your benefit, and insert a variety of compelling stories of other patients who have written me during this journey. There is much to gain from the life experiences of other Parkinson's or Parkinson's Plus patients and their care giving spouses or family members. I will put all of this in a context of my individual faith in God, which has been the sustaining force that has enabled me to deal with the impact of a neuro-degenerative disease with hope and dignity.

Chapter One
Why Me? My Story of Diagnosis

I AM ASSUMING YOU OR a loved one has recently found out they have Parkinson's Disease or a similar Parkinson's-like condition that has created a great need for information on how to go on with your life. Parkinson's Disease or Parkinson's Plus is not the end, nor would I go as far as to call living with one of these diseases a beginning. Let's face it—this situation you find yourself in is not fun and is not particularly inspiring. I do know, as an individual that has just completed my first year of dealing with the decline which results from the neurodegenerative qualities of Parkinson's Plus syndrome, that the effects represent a tremendous blow to the patient's future plans and expectations for his or her life. In order to make some important decisions about telling your family, what to say to the boss, how to adjust your expectations for your career and answering the question of finances that have gripped your life, you will need as much information as you can find.

This book is going to be a valuable source of information on facing the condition you now find yourself with, on a human level, if not to some degree, on a technical one. I will explain exactly what Parkinson's Disease and Parkinson's Plus conditions are, and describe the resulting serious disabilities affecting both body and mind. I will tell you my story, in brief, in order to give you an idea of who I am and also to give you an understanding of the way I have been affected, personally. I hope to support you by both giving you information that will assist you with understanding the disease, and by providing you with the opportunity to identify with me and others who face similar disappointments and challenges. The fact that I am not a medical doctor, but rather a patient whose only expertise in dealing with this condition is that which I have derived by personal experience and research of my own, is something I want to make clear from the beginning. The thought is that this "patient's perspective" would give me a unique viewpoint that I hope that you will find interesting, if not beneficial.

Introduction to My Story

The following is a chronological, personal description of the signs and symptoms that I was experiencing during the time just prior to my seeing a neurologist for the first time. If I had been aware of these conditions previous to being affected, they may have acted as guideposts that indicated the Parkinson's Plus syndrome was coming on and would eventually appear in living color many years later. I have pieced together the story of these earliest signs and explained how these preceding years merged with the diagnostic process that followed.

I was a healthy, athletic person most of my life, with several injuries resulting from sports and other work-related injuries. I had torn knee ligaments, tendonitis in my left knee, badly sprained ankles on both sides, and above all, serious back injuries, beginning with sophomore football in high school. It seems that once I injured my back in the summer I turned 15, it was a recurring problem again and again. I repeatedly exacerbated the problem every time I lifted heavy furniture, or landed wrong after jumping for a rebound in basketball. My road running hobby by my late 20's seemed to contribute to a chronic and painful lumbar condition. By my 30th birthday, while I was teaching in my fifth year and finishing up my master's degree, and after severe pain and obvious disc injuries, I sought out care for the unbearable discomfort I was experiencing. This pain had made it difficult to walk, and interfered with the important things in life, such as picking up my small sons, and my professional responsibilities as a teacher and program coordinator in public schools. This back trouble made it nearly impossible to even think of playing golf, softball, basketball or continuing with my hobby of distance running.

Early Back Troubles

I had my first of three back surgeries in 1986 and returned to work six weeks later with residual pain and a sense that I would never be quite the same again. I healed over time, and eventually returned to occasional golf, and even running for fitness, for several years. But by 1995, my back pain became more serious than ever in my history, and I began to lose proper nerve function in my left leg. I was walking with a flopping left foot, that formally was labeled, "drop foot." By the time I went through all of the hoops and tests, several months had passed leaving me with permanent scarring on my spinal nerves from the constant pressure of ruptured discs that had spilled into my spinal column. These severe injuries had produced nerve pinching in my lower back that immobilized me and resulted in excruciatingly painful burning and shock sensations in both feet. I was experiencing much loss of feeling in my left foot and ankle, in particular. In spite of the pain, I worked daily, relying on a cane to walk any significant distance of a half block or more.

I had my second lower lumbar operation in the summer of 1995 and took three months to recover enough to return to my principal role at a large elementary school. Because of the residual effects of the surgery itself, which was very intrusive and required the removal of scar tissue and bone that was compressing nerve roots traveling to my left leg, I was somewhat permanently disabled. I thank God that at the early age of 40 years I was in my fifth year as a school administrator and was able to fully handle the responsibilities that I had, from a physical standpoint. The classroom would have been very difficult for me at this time, due to the need to bend over student desks and remain standing for extended periods. This surgery was badly timed in that I had finally completed production of my first CD, entitled, "A Long Time Comin'" and it limited my physical ability needed to perform and promote it as an independent music project that I had so long dreamed of creating. This period preceded my next professional assignment as principal at a middle school with 1500 students, in the school year, 1996–1997.

Fusion

My second back surgery had a sequel. In 1999 I went back under the knife to have two levels of my lower lumbar fused, and this procedure also included more decompression of nerve roots. In addition, bone was removed from my upper, right hip to be placed between the two spaces where two lumbar discs were removed in order to provide what I would call an organic fusion, absent of metal, screws or other hardware. I saw it as a very positive aspect that my outstanding orthopedic surgeon was able to create a durable fusion of this part of my back without metals and other foreign bodies that would have surely needed to be removed. This surgery resulted in a very solid and permanent strength in my lower back and removed the potential for a recurrence later in my life. I had permanent limitations with sports that I have dearly missed, I walked with a permanent limp, had permanent nerve damage, but looking back now, I realize

I was able to work another eight years without ever taking a single day off to rest or recover from back pain. Part of that was my strength and sense of responsibility, but I also give my great surgeon who handled both the second and third back surgeries much credit for giving me the ability to continue providing for my family.

To this day, if it were a question of my back interfering with work, I would have been able to carry out my duties in my last position of assistant superintendent of personnel in a growing school district. I have to say though, the main reason I could go on was that I was a very tough and determined person, and my threshold for enduring pain was very, very high. Many would have gone on permanent disability by this point in my personal history, at the young age of 44. God was good to me in that He saw me through these years of pain and physical loss, giving me a sense of purpose and confidence.

What Is Shaking?

Now, after this surgery, in 1999, I first notice what I thought were tremors. When I would sit in my office having a conference with one of my teachers, I would see a small, repetitive trembling of my hand. I passed it off for years as the result of low blood sugar or too much caffeine, a reasonable reaction, since I was looking to downplay this sign. At home I began to spot the tiniest movement of my face and chin, as I would stare into the mirror to shave or trim my beard. I remember thinking, "Is that really my head shaking or am I imagining it?" I would on occasion show my wife, but neither of us was concerned and I thought it might be a nerve problem resulting from the prolonged time under anesthesia during back surgeries. The point is, I was healthy enough and this fine, barely noticeable tremor didn't interfere with anything I was doing, so I kept on working as a principal as though nothing was bothering me.

I advanced my career, went back to school to get a doctorate degree in education from La Sierra University, in Riverside, California, and I subsequently applied for a district office position. During this pursuit of the district office I had always dreamed of in the personnel area of school district leadership, I was completely unaware and unconcerned about any signs that I had of Parkinsonism. Because I had no knowledge at that time that led me to believe that something was happening in my brain that would eventually blossom into a serious condition, I went on as if these fine trembling sensations were merely individual peculiarities that came with my aging process. As far back as 2003, right after graduating and being selected for the district level position as director of personnel services in a public school district in the Inland Empire of Southern California, I can remember in hindsight having several initial signs, none of which drove me to the doctor. At the time, I attributed these signs to my back surgeries and all of my physical problems seemed to stem from these three, serious spinal operations.

I gave my all and hustled all day in the office, but I was lethargic and lacked energy when I would arrive home from a 12-hour day in the office, which included a 30-minute commute both ways. In the years preceding this time in my life, when I arrived home from work, I was the type to work in the yard, go shopping with my wife, or play catch with my sons. But in 2003, I started a pattern of eating dinner, sitting for hours at a time and falling asleep in my chair, never to return to the land of the living for the rest of the evening. Quietly, my wife was becoming concerned. When we walked together, I who had always been a fast paced and competitive walker, lagged behind, and as she explains now that things have come out about my disease, she wondered why no matter how she slowed her pace to benefit me, I would only go more slowly and remain behind her around the entire community trail on which we walked.

I began to have stiffness in my ankles and feet, and rose slowly from a chair with a very stiff and awkward walk as I would take the first ten or fifteen steps. I had no energy, had frequent head aches in my eyes, some blurring of vision and never felt like I could get my glasses prescribed right. I had a great deal of stiffness in my feet and ankles in the fall of 2004, and it would take a while after getting up from a chair for my ankles to start bending and moving.

Meanwhile, I had complaints of feeling lightheaded and walking into doorways, with my shoulder banging into the door post quite frequently. Each day, my wife and I would pray in the garage, before my departure. She got into the habit of holding my shoulders because when I closed my eyes to pray I would rock back and forth, and sway in a way that led Karrie to think I might fall. Again, we just attributed this to balance issues stemming from nerve problems from my back surgeries and injuries. We were not concerned because I was still putting in 12-hour days on the road and in the office.

Then, in the summer of 2005, my head-nodding tremor began to be more prominent, but still only appeared when I was sitting still, thus months later it would be labeled a "resting tremor." This was the most obvious and pronounced symptom I had that those at work and in my family could identify as "the problem." I would notice it most when I was in a conference in my office, listening to an employee or client. I would feel as though I was nodding in agreement, but then I would not stop nodding "yes," as though my head and neck could not stop this motion. On a few occasions, I asked a colleague if they were able to see my head bobbing or if they noticed it. Rarely did anyone else see anything. Two years before, my wife, Karrie, would indicate that she was not sure, but that she thought if I had a concern, I "should go to the doctor." Finally, Karrie was noticing it while we were in the family room at night watching television. In the late spring of 2005, she indicated that she was able to see it and it was pronounced enough for her to be worried about what it might mean. Two months later, in August of 2005, I made an appointment to go see my primary care doctor.

First Time at the Doctor's Office

This primary care doctor agreed that something was going on, that it was Parkinsonian in nature, and referred me to a neurologist to have further tests. He said it could be Parkinson's Disease or Essential Tremor, but he wanted the specialist to make that determination. He told me, that my "head wasn't going to fall off, so stop worrying so much." He gave me a choice of neurologists, and I selected the one that was easier to schedule, a decision I regretted later. There was a neurologist he recommended but it would take two months to get in to see him. I went to the first neurologist and after two visits he declared I had Dystonia. I had an MRI with no significant findings, and my blood was tested for every obvious serious illness, including Wilson's Disease, Mad Cow Disease, and Multiple Sclerosis, and there were no findings. He prescribed Levodopa/Carbidopa, and eventually added Comtan, which collectively seemed to work well to calm my head tremor and whole left arm that had begun to shake. These drugs would give me relief for up to two hours, but the question persisted about what form of Parkinsonism I had, although this neurologist clearly declared that I had a Parkinsonian condition.

A Faster Progression

Then all hell broke lose. My condition began to progress so rapidly that it was really baffling. I started having shaking in both arms and my trunk trembled at all times, particularly when at rest. By October I was noticing I had some trouble forming words and I would notice my mouth was struggling to keep up when I talked. I coughed and sputtered often when I ate or drank. By November of 2005, my legs began to shake, and if standing in one place, I had trouble keeping my knees from swaying from side-to-side. Along with the swaying, my mouth was beginning to draw down into a frown and I could feel my chin trembling.

By December I began to struggle to control my legs when I walked. I was on a holiday outing with my family, including my wife, grown children and my mother. I was not coordinated and my arms did not swing in sync. It was a very scary moment when I realized that I had to sit down and wait for my family to finish walking on the light displays along the boardwalk of a costal city an hour from our home. My legs felt as though they were foreign to me and I had the sense that if I continued to walk in the dim light of that boardwalk along the canal, I would surely fall on the concrete.

My hands, by January 2006, had chronic, constant tremors. I began to notice whenever I put my arm around my wife or held her hand, I would have an unstoppable intention tremor. I was having times when my thinking would become confused, for lack of a better way of putting it. I returned to the original primary care physician and I requested that I be referred to a second neurologist to deal with the many questions I was amassing and the unusually fast progression of symptoms. The second and highly recommended neurologist, Dr. N, was outstanding and began to address our concerns directly and with great compassion, as well as professionalism. Keep in mind though, I didn't see Dr. N until February of 2006, five months after my first complaint to our primary care physician.

I now walked with a cane anywhere I went on foot outside of the house. I needed to be taken home from work twice in December 2005 and another time in January 2006. This is also when I began to notice my speech getting worse, and I was struggling with my eyelids wanting to close involuntarily during each period of tremors. Eventually, my eyes starting alternating between lid closure to opening so wide they were bugging out, and my mouth went into a grimace when my eyes would assume this alarmed appearance.

I had trouble with decisions and slowed responses to the questions my wife posed, such as whether or not I wanted to go shopping with her. It had reached a point where the new neurologist was doing an excellent job of investigating my case, and he ordered a number of tests, including a spinal tap to test for Multiple Sclerosis and Mad Cow's disease. I had a Positron Emissions Topography (PET) to look for signs of Alzheimer's, and the results were negative for Alzheimer's. However, the radiologist noticed just a bit of atrophy in the left Frontal Lobe. Incidentally, getting a PET scan was something that took an appeal through the medical board of our medical clinic. I must say, the individual who served as the appeal representative that worked for the medical insurance carrier was very helpful and fair. I believe it was because of her compassion that the PET scan was finally granted, even though the results could be defined as inconclusive for the most part.

Neuro-Psychological Testing

A neuro-psychologist, Dr. P tested me for weeks in the late winter and spring of 2006, and determined that I had deficits in working memory, not "long-term" memory. He stated that I had difficulty with attention and memory of discussions from approximately 20 minutes earlier. He determined that there were signs that could lead to a form of dementia that subtly affected memory and language, but weren't attributable to an Alzheimer's condition. What the neuro-psychologist found were signs of cognitive effects, tantamount to a case of Parkinson's Disease. I was very fortunate to be referred to Dr. P due to his empathetic style and years of experience testing patients with Parkinson's symptoms for cognitive function issues.

In late February, Dr. N indicated I should stop driving due to issues with coordination and reflexes, and asked me to take a six-month sabbatical from my career. This was a shocking turn of events. I had no idea at the time that I would never be able to return to either of these vital activities that gave me a sense of usefulness and purpose, every day. I never knew how I took the freedom and privilege of driving for granted, let alone the value that my professional role had in giving me a place to use the talents God had given me to help guide and shape people's lives toward successful personal development. I went from a school district, cabinet-level administrative post (having a background as a school principal) with a doctorate degree (Ed.D.) completed in 2003, to the point of not being able to drive or deal with the verbal demands of my position. To make matters worse, my difficulty walking with any rhythm and coordination, was getting worse by the week.

During the Spring of 2006, I was declared 100% permanently disabled and began the process of applying for the state teacher's retirement disability pension. In the ensuing months, I began to have more and more difficulties with my eyes. They were either bugged out and possessed a shocked expression, accompanied by my mouth pulling open and down on one side, or my eyes had a sensation as though the muscles were pulling them up, or up and down, in circular motions. This caused eye pain and made it difficult to focus on an object or person that I wanted to see.

Disability and No Wheels

Dr. N was concerned about how unsteady my walk had become and the constant tremors that were affecting my entire body. These signs, including the balance issues, eye movement difficulties, cognitive affects, speech issues, bradykinesia (involuntarily slow movements) and overall instability of my posture, led to his concern and resulted in the thorough battery of medical tests he pursued. My neurologist concluded that I had a form of Parkinsonism that would be defined better as my various symptoms "emerged," or basically became worse and more pronounced. He referred to it technically as an "Extrapyramidal Disorder" and an "Abnormal, Involuntary Movement Disorder."

In May 2006, with all of the knowledge derived from the neuro-psychological testing report and his own clinical observations, my neurologist further defined my condition as a Parkinsonism Plus and stated it could be either Shy Drager Syndrome or Progressive Supranuclear Palsy. In the ensuing months after the spring of 2006, my eye movement difficulties grew in severity, limiting my up and down, and right and left movements. Additionally, my hands and forearms were developing a weak and shaky feeling, more and more, while my fine dexterity was being impacted gradually. This took the form of dropping forks, and breaking drinking glasses, along with a slightly more noticeable difficulty in squeezing my guitar neck when I would play a bar chord.

Parkinson's Plus

Later, in the spring of 2007, my neurologist indicated that the form of Parkinson's Plus I was most likely to have was Progressive Supranuclear Palsy. My walking has limited me to a cane on any walks beyond my front door, and I require a wheel chair or mobility scooter for any walking beyond a single block, such as shopping or sight seeing. Travel requires a scooter on a lift attached to our mini-van so that my wife and I are able to go together to any shops or sight seeing locations. I choke at times when swallowing, requiring me to cough for 20 minutes to clear my airway of small, irritating particles or liquid. My throat muscles are softening and the movement difficulties that affect other parts of my body, are also affecting my swallowing apparatus, the strength of my voice and my eye lids.

Above, all else, I feel dizzy and off balance more and more, and I tend to tip over or fall back into a chair, so I must think about every move I make to be sure I am not jeopardizing my safety. I am having cognitive changes that cause me to forget occurrences from less than 15 and up to 60 minutes earlier. I have difficulty speaking with fluency when my medications are wearing off, and, at times, I have a spastic quality to my speech which makes me sound a bit complacent or lacking in voice dynamics. It is very frustrating and noticeable for me as a strong communicator throughout my life, although close friends and family don't find it to be a hindrance or very noticeable.

My wife, Karrie, would say that she is much more able to detect the speech difficulty than others. It is as though it takes me a while to get started when asked a question or if I go to interject an idea in a conversation. After starting to speak, I frequently don't get to finish because either people aren't hearing me or they thought I was finished with my first four-word phrase. Often, I am just getting started and I have to pause for a moment to locate my next idea and by then, things have moved on and it is too late to bother. It is an isolating feeling that is caused by no one outside of myself, but makes me feel as though my purpose for interacting with others is slipping away. I find that I am less inclined to want to speak in certain situations now.

My face has reached a point of being more and more masked, with my eyes blinking much, much less than ever before, and they also tend to pop open, giving me a shocked expression. My mouth will either be in a frown or a drawn and grimaced shape. The medications I take, or have taken, including Sinemet, Artane and Azilect all help these above symptoms. At times, because of these medications, I am much more able to speak, move with some ease, force a smile and shake less. I am not helped with walking difficulty or "eye hang-ups," as my neurologist calls them, much at all by these Parkinson's drugs. However, Sinemet and Artane, along with Azilect, seem to lift my mood and improve my outlook considerably. I will even feel renewed energy for the time the meds are working. Sinemet wears off in approximately two hours, and I experience dyskinesia in the form of writhing and random movements of my head, harms, hands and feet, as the dopamine levels in my brain drop off.

I am more and more aware of a loss of fine motor use of my hands, and I fear that I will have difficulty with guitar playing, which is something I am not prepared to accept. This activity (guitar playing) has always been second nature and required no strain at all. I plan to play on and on, ignoring the cramping pain in my wrists or the slight change in coordination or muscle strength. I refuse to let go of my music, as it has been with me since the age of seven. My cognitive functioning is a problem I could not see coming, nor do I plan to give in to that possible decline. I read as much as I can, write something on the computer every day and work on memorizing new songs to sing as often as I can find the words and chords on free online sources.

My Blessings

My wife has developed systems, such as a white board on which events on the daily calendar are listed and she frequently tries to get me involved in errands and outings by giving me choices of where to go and when. Her efforts, positive attitude, and kind words all lift me and are as medicinal as any other treatment I experience. I am a blessed man, in spite of all of these challenges and difficulties. My three adult sons and daughter-in-law are very special to me and I find great satisfaction in family outings or meals. We get together frequently and are a very close family. I am not sure what the future will hold, but I will keep fighting by participating in church, support groups, and writing my online blog. Eventually, I determined to write this book focusing on the challenges I have faced and overcome while on this medical journey. In the meantime, every day is a gift and I plan to live each one to its fullest.

My Condition Now

I can't often keep a gaze at a person talking with me, as I subconsciously look at the table or off in the distance. Sometimes my eyes cross and everything goes to two images. My hands are becoming more and more awkward in curling postures and they feel like I am losing control over them slowly. They feel light, weak and strange. Sometimes I have to correct my typing again and again.

My toes curl up when I put up my feet while sitting in my recliner. When I sit at the table they tap up and down inside my shoes in a steady tremor. I am taking Sinemet four times a day and Artane two administrations per day. I have depression, anxiety and difficulty sleeping.

In a short two-year timeframe I became permanently disabled from my thirty-year career as an educator, and that fact is quite disappointing. I feel so different from the other Parkinson's Disease patients, who in the first several years, typically have a hand that shakes, but they are functioning and driving. I am only 53, but I feel like I am going down hill much more quickly than other patients in our support group, including some that are 20 or more years older than me. This is, presumably, due to the fact that my condition is Parkinson's Plus, not idiopathic Parkinson's Disease.

My eyes have become much more of an issue. In addition, I frequently lose my balance and have caught myself before tragically falling on a number of occasions. I have actually slipped or fallen only twice, although I have felt myself get light-headed enough to partially black out and go to my knees several times in recent weeks. I never actually have gone completely out, but I have felt close to it and grabbed the counter several times.

As mentioned above, I take a new drug called Azilect, which has an alternate name, Rasageline. This medicine, approved by the Food and Drug Administration in May of 2006, is said to have a neuro-protective ability and could as a result, potentially slow the progression or presumed brain cell loss. I now go to Dr. N, the neurologist, every three months and there are no more tests that need to be run, in the foreseeable future, other than periodic MRI's and psychological testing. That is a nice place to be in many ways, but still unresolved are the questions so many of us facing a serious bout with Parkinsonism face, which are, "When will the diagnosis be complete? Which form of Parkinson's Plus will I end up having?" Dr. N used the analogy of a flower. He explained, your condition "hasn't blossomed yet" in order to indicate exactly which form I have, Progressive Supranuclear Palsy or Multiple Systems Atrophy (also referred to as Shy Drager).

In order to explain the differences between these two categories of PD Plus, and to lay the ground work for the rest of the information I provide in this book, in my next chapter I will proceed to outline the hallmark symptoms of Parkinson's Disease, followed by the explanation of what Parkinson's Plus is by definition. Just to touch on it, Parkinson's Plus is an atypical form of P.D., with other complications. Stay tuned for more in coming chapters.

Chapter Two

Symptoms of Parkinson's Disease

PARKINSON'S IS A DISEASE that affects the movement center of the brain, known as the Basal Ganglia. Within the Basal Ganglia, the Substantia Nigra is gradually losing cells that produce a neuro-transmitter known as dopamine. Dopamine interacts with acetylcholine, and together they create proper, coordinated movements. With the loss of dopamine, which is an ever increasing problem in Parkinson's Disease, tremors, stiffness, coordination problems, and slow movements ensue. Parkinson's Disease is a progressive disorder, which means these changes grow worse over time and are chronic in nature, meaning it is not able to be arrested. Over time, the Parkinson's Disease patient will have more and more difficulty with movement and the condition will eventually progress to the point of the patient freezing when medications are worn off. I have outlined the major symptoms of Parkinson's Disease below.

Tremor

There are a variety of tremor types, including intention tremor, postural tremor, but the typical and most prevalent type is known as resting tremor. This tremor is characterized by an involuntary, rhythmic movement of an affected limb (hand, foot, arm, chin, lip, or head) and occurs during a time of rest. The more still the patient becomes the more likely the resting tremor is to be produced, involuntarily. Approximately 30% of all Parkinson's patients do not have a tremor of any kind.

Bradykinesia

The slowness in initiating movements or motor functions is another of the primary or classic symptoms of Parkinson's Disease. It consists of slowed walking gait, hand movements, functions of the mouth (including speech), blinking or swallowing mechanism.

Rigidity

A hallmark symptom of Parkinson's Disease is the resulting stiffness or rigidity. This describes the poverty of movement related to the increased muscle tone resulting from the effects of P.D. This stiffness is evident when attempting to move an arm, leg, neck or other affected limbs or joints.

Balance Problems

Typically, as the disease progresses, the patient will begin to face difficulty with overall balance and walking gait disturbances. This results from a loss of postural reflexes and brings about poor posture and balance. The walking pattern becomes increasingly restricted to smaller steps and may give the appearance of marching. Turning becomes increasingly more deliberate and is referred to as turning en block. The patient will eventually struggle to walk and have an increased potential to fall. This will typically begin on one side and eventually progress to the other, as well. In addition, the tendency to freeze in one place contributes to the balance issues leading to frequent falls. Patients also may begin walking with a series of quick, small steps as if hurrying forward to keep balance, a practice known as festinating.

Additional Symptoms

Parkinson's Disease is not limited to tremor, which is the recognizable problem most in society think defines it as a disease. Other symptoms add to its severity, and in reality cause as much or more difficulty performing daily tasks or continuing to function in a profession or maintaining favorite activities. Some of these symptoms are more subtle, but nonetheless, may be both serious and painful to experience. Each patient will have varying numbers of these symptoms and will be impacted more or less severely, depending on the progression of the individual illness. Parkinson's symptoms appear in no particular order, and at varying rates. Some individuals have a faster progression of symptoms and others are fortunate to have the disease progress very slowly. In my case, by the time I became aware of the tremors, I began to progress very rapidly and was unable to continue in my career within seven months of my first recognition of the effects of my Extrapyramidal Disorder, which is at least similar to Parkinson's Disease. This list is inclusive of as many symptoms as could be found, but it may not include all of the possibilities:

- Fatigue or general malaise

- Trembling

- Difficulty arising from a seated position

- Lowered voice volume (dysarthria)

- Small, cramped, spidery handwriting

- Losing track of a word or thought

- Irritability or sadness for no apparent reason

- Lack of expression in the face (reduced blinking, smiling)

- Lack of animation

- Remaining in a certain position for long period of time

- Unable to normally move an arm or leg

Secondary Symptoms

Secondary symptoms are no less difficult and should not be viewed as insignificant. Secondary indicates that they are not found in a consistent manner with each patient, but are frequently observed clinically.

- Depression

- Dementia (resulting in cognitive difficulties, particularly with short term or working memory)

- Difficulty with speaking

- Emotional changes (increased fearfulness and insecurity)

- Memory loss and slowed thinking

- Difficulty with drooling, swallowing and chewing

- Urinary problems or constipation

- Skin problems

- Sleep problems

The symptoms of Parkinson's disease may resemble other conditions or medical problems. Always consult your physician for a diagnosis.

Two of the four categories of primary Parkinson's Disease symptoms listed at the beginning of this section are necessary to be present in order to be diagnosed with the disease. Moreover, in many cases three of four would be easily observed at the time of diagnosis. It is important to note that as I have become more knowledgeable about this illness, I find that there are frequently exceptions as no two cases are exactly alike. It is very naïve to believe that Parkinson's Disease is easily identifiable or simple to confirm. There are those who have no tremor (30%) and yet tremor is the most likely first symptom to be noticed and often leads to the first visit to the doctor to inquire, "What is going on with me?" Be very careful to not read any list such as this and think that you can make an absolute diagnosis or assumption about a condition as complex as this one. You will need an expert neurologist or movement disorder specialist taking the necessary steps to determine the degree to which these primary and secondary symptoms are present in order to make an absolute diagnosis. These are included in this book with the intent of serving as guidelines or information from a patient perspective, thus leading to an appointment with a qualified physician.

Another important point to remember is that a newly diagnosed Parkinson's patient does not start out with the full gamut of the disease. Sometimes a patient will have the appearance of a dominant tremor condition or instead, the patient may exhibit a great deal of stiffness and slowness. When these appear in isolation and with no other initial symptoms, it would result in more difficulty in diagnosing Parkinson's Disease early in the onset of the condition. This does not mean an individual does not have Parkinson's, it merely indicates that the final determination is difficult at that moment and more time may be needed to observe and evaluate the changes that will take place later in the course of the disease. *I can't emphasis enough the importance of seeing a neurologist as soon as you become aware of these primary or secondary symptoms.*

Parkinson's Plus

Sometimes other conditions share similar symptoms and mimic Parkinson's Disease. One group of these conditions are known as Parkinson's Plus and differ in that they meet the following criteria: 1) have a much more rapid onset, 2) are not as responsive to Levodopa therapy 3) the condition presents as bilateral rather than unilateral as is found in idiopathic Parkinson's Disease, and 4) the patient will exhibit serious balance, gait, speech, swallowing or eye movement problems early in the disease onset.

Parkinsonism Plus Syndrome is a group of degenerative neurological conditions, which differ from Parkinson's Disease in specific clinical features, such as: a poor response to Levodopa, distinctive physical and neurological symptoms not necessarily found in Parkinson's Disease, and a shorter term life expectancy. Additional symptomatic differences that are often observed include, but are not limited to, the following: infrequent or atypical tremor, prominent muscular rigidity, pronounced bradykinesia (or slowed movement), early onset of postural instability, supranuclear gaze palsy (difficulty with eye movements and/or looking down), earlier autonomic failure, Cerebellar signs (such as a severe lack of coordination of movements), alien limb phenomenon, apraxia and prominent early cognitive disorders that may occur more frequently. Progressive Supranuclear palsy (PSP), Multiple System Atrophy, Corticobasal Ganglionic Degeneration and Dementia with Lewy Body disease (DLB) are the most common conditions known as Parkinson's Plus disorders.

In recent years it has become apparent to the medical community that it is difficult to distinguish some variants of these Parkinson's Plus conditions from each other. The term Multiple Systems Atrophy is used to describe three different specific conditions that may overlap in some cases: Shy Drager Syndrome, Striato-Nigral Degeneration, and Olivopontocerebellar Atrophy.

However, unusual presentations and combinations of varying complications make the diagnosis more difficult. In my case, Parkinson's Plus syndrome was as specific a diagnosis as could be achieved given the data and observable symptoms my neurologist had to go on. In time, it will become apparent whether my condition should be defined as Progressive Supranuclear Palsy, Multiple Systems Atrophy or another syndrome. It is also apparent to me, from my research in books and online sources, that there are individuals who have a hybrid condition, which includes two or more groups of symptoms such as Parkinson's and Lou Gehrig's Disease, as an example.

> "Will shall be the sterner, heart the bolder, spirit the greater as our strength lessens."
> –from the Anglo-Saxon "Battle of Maldon," as quoted in THE INKLINGS, written by Humprey Carpenter (Houghton Mifflin, Boston, 1979). This was a quote of the great writer C.S. Lewis as he was heard referencing this piece in conversation.

Chapter Three

The Parkinson's Plus Conditions – A User Friendly Explanation

IN THIS CHAPTER, I will outline the salient features and symptoms of various Parkinson's Plus diseases. I will purposefully write these from a lay-person, patient perspective. It is also fair to point out that I am not experiencing Parkinson's Plus in a vacuum, as I can not separate the person I am from my efforts in this book.

User Friendly Approach

As an individual who has spent 30 years of my life working in the educational arena as an instructional assistant, classroom teacher, school site principal, district office administrator and adjunct professor of graduate school courses, I will try to write in a way that emphasizes an understanding of the information that will be transferable to a family and friend context. This way, those who use this book as a reference will find it more meaningful in helping others to get a better idea of what these diseases are about, in the way they affect real people, not "medical subjects." Later in this book I will contrast Parkinson's Plus with Parkinson's Disease, using my own case as an example. Much of the confusion I see in communicating this information is related to the perception that these are all just "fancy names for Parkinson's Disease," as a well-meaning friend stated on one occasion.

What are The Parkinson's Plus Syndromes?

As a foundation for this first disease I will write about, Progressive Supranuclear Palsy, let me remind the reader that Parkinson's Plus conditions, which include both Multiple Systems Atrophy (MSA has three subtypes) and PSP, are conditions which involve the degeneration of the Basal Ganglia, which is the movement center of the brain. Parkinson's and Parkinson's Plus, will generally affect this part of the brain in that both will have a loss of the cells in this area governing movement, leading to a lack of dopamine. Dopamine is required by the brain in order to bring about normal and properly coordinated movements. This lack of dopamine causes the symptoms of Parkinson's that are generally included in Parkinson's Plus, such as tremors, postural instability (balance difficulty), rigidity and slowness of movement (bradykinesia). To clarify further: although the Parkinson's Plus diseases typically have some aspects of these symptoms resulting from dopamine loss, Parkinson's Plus is not merely another name for Parkinson's Disease or a more serious version, but it is a disease which has the Parkinson's symptoms plus other serious conditions.

Depending on the additional areas of the brain which are degenerating, other symptoms appear which are named for their particular resulting conditions. Some are more Parkinson's-like, such as Corticobasal Ganglionic Degeneration and Striato-Nigral Degeneration, while others are more focused on cognitive difficulties such as Dementia with Lewy Bodies, and still others reflect greater difficulty with walking and standing balance, or mobility, namely Olivopontocerebellar Atrophy

(OPCA) and Progressive Supranuclear Palsy. Additionally, there are others that affect eye movements (PSP and OPCA), while another is focused on autonomic systems, such as the regulation of blood pressure, and bowel and bladder functions as found in the MSA subtype, Shy Drager Syndrome.

All typically affect speech, swallowing, cognition, balance, abnormal movements, slowness of movement, and walking difficulty, to some degree or another. These overlapping signs make the diagnostic process very complex, and thus suggest that a movement disorder specialist be seen in order to make an early diagnosis to determine the best course of treatment.

Progressive Supranuclear Palsy

My first topic will be Progressive Supranuclear Palsy (PSP), a condition that does not respond well to drugs used to treat Parkinson's-like symptoms. Difficulty in controlling eye movements is one symptom which makes PSP distinct from the Multiple Systems Atrophy diseases, such as Corticobasal Ganglionic Degeneration, Striato-Nigral Degeneration, Olivopontocerebellar Atrophy, Dementia with Lewy Bodies, and Shy Drager Syndrome.

PSP causes the eyes to gradually lose their ability to move, particularly up and down. This lack of eye movement causes difficulty for the patient to see where he or she is going, and interferes with reading and eating. The "dirty tie sign" is the name given to the effect this difficulty in looking down causes. The range of motion of a PSP patient's eyes in looking down is limited, leading to frequent spills on clothes, thus the reference to the soiling of the traditional neck-tie. Also, swallowing becomes problematic due to the weaker movements of the mouth, tongue and throat. Patients need to be encouraged to eat with great care and a speech therapist is helpful in guiding the patient in this regard.

As swallowing becomes a more serious issue, the patient will cough during or after eating. The inability to control the swallowing apparatus will often lead to aspiration pneumonia late in the course of the illness. A feeding tube may eventually be necessary to avoid serious complications that could threaten the life of the PSP patient. Problems with bladder and bowel control, although a primary symptom found in Shy Drager Syndrome, does often trouble the PSP patient, and may become quite severe over time.

Although this illness is often confused with Parkinson's Disease, the resting tremor of Parkinson's is seen much less often, although it may occur. The disease appears as early as a patient's 40's, although it is more common in the 60's. Cases involving men are more prevalent than women, and PSP accounts for five percent of the patient's complaining of Parkinsonism at medical facilities dealing with neurological diseases. Changes in the protein *tau* lead to neural degeneration. These changes lead to an aggregation of fibrillar polymers, known as "taupathies." Patients live an average of 10 years after diagnosis, but this is an approximation. Dr. P, my neuro-psychologist, explained that an individual's circumstances—quality of treatment, family and friend support network, age, overall health prior to disease onset, home environment, and mental outlook—all may contribute to a better prognosis. I would add that, in my personal opinion, faith in God plays an important role in the health of the Parkinson's Plus patient and the spiritual perspective is very beneficial, also possibly enhancing longevity.

Visual Succades and Eye Movement Difficulties

In addition to eye movements being limited in their up and down motion, the ability of the eyes to pursue moving objects develops a glitch causing a delay in the actual tracking of the eyes horizontally. This may be found when the neurologist holds a pen light and moves it slowly from left to right, and back to center. The eyes will show signs of difficulty in smoothly making this pursuit. Individuals with PSP will often not make eye contact as you would normally expect when facing someone in conversation. This individual is not ignoring you, but rather has trouble neurologically in forcing the eyes to fix on you as the speaker. It is more comfortable, I know from experience, to gaze off to the side of the person speaking.

The eyes may also have a Dystonia of the eyelids called "blepharospasm", referring to the eyes closing involuntarily, temporarily, and in some cases for a longer and more debilitating period of time, requiring some type of treatment to prevent loss of sight. A PSP patient will sometimes see double images or have difficulty focusing on a fixed point. It is also common for PSP patients to have a wide-eyed stare resulting from the eyelids being forced open, coupled with reduced blinking, which leads to problems with dry and irritated eyes. Sensitivity to light is often an increasingly troubling issue, as is the gradual reduction of the peripheral field of vision.

Walking Gait Difficulty

Progressive Supranuclear Palsy causes the patient to have difficulty coordinating the walking gait, in addition to a stiff-legged walk and balance difficulty. This gait instability will often result in falls, sometimes early in the course of illness. Falling is ultimately a very serious symptom of this disease and will become a reason for the patient to become permanently wheelchair bound. This problem occurs to different levels of severity and at varying rates of onset in each patient.

No two PSP patients have exactly the same course of onset of any of the various symptoms I am describing. This is due to a variety of factors such as age, overall initial health at time of onset and environmental aspects such as physical layout of the home and the degree of assistance from a care giver and or family member. The variance in amount of falling occurrences, and/or resulting injury, will depend on the individual circumstances. The increasing inability to move the eyes to a downward position, will contribute to difficulty walking with coordination. This will make walking on stairs a very serious consideration, if not virtually impossible to accomplish for some patients.

Axial Rigidity

While rigidity is a factor in Parkinson's-like illnesses, including generally all Parkinson's Plus conditions listed earlier in this article, PSP will cause a stiffness focused most severely on the neck and spine, making it difficult to turn easily and causing postural instability contributing to a progressive loss of balance. This condition, known as axial rigidity, results in a great deal of cramping and stiffness. Arms and hands assume awkward positions and the fingers may tend to close tightly in the palms. The toes will tend to turn up or down as the feet are also affected by the stiffening that accompanies parkinsonism. Worrisome neck pain is often an early symptom, but not initially recognized as related to PSP since this condition is often present in other injuries or diseases. Often the neck will be hyper-extended in an upward position, adding to vision difficulties and creating great discomfort.

Dysarthria

In PSP, speech is seriously affected. Early in the course of the illness, a patient, thought to have Parkinson's Disease, will begin to have balance difficulties, stiffness and rigidity of the spine and neck and, the speech will begin to become slurred or lack volume. Speech is affected both physically, due to the affects of the disease bringing about slowed movements, but also due to the cognitive aspects that are involved in the illness. Patients will have difficulty responding to questions or trouble remembering the topic, leading to the perception that they are not aware of what is happening around them. This assumption is not necessarily true, but rather is a serious aspect of the illness and the patient appreciates patience as they work to organize their thoughts and coordinate their mouth to reply or explain their request. In time, PSP will in many cases lead to the patient's inability to speak at all.

Emotional and Cognitive Difficulties

Emotionally, most PSP patients will exhibit depression, because of the effect of the disease on neurotransmitters in the brain that relate to emotions and moods. PSP patients will often be prescribed some form of anti-depressant or anti-psychotic drugs to deal with these difficulties. The patient's personality may appear to have changed before noticing other symptoms that lead to a visit to the doctor, and their behavior may be unlike the person to which friends and family were accustomed. For example, the patient may exhibit a loss of interest in ordinary pleasurable activities or demonstrate increased irritability. PSP also has cognitive effects, and will potentially lead to mild or more serious dementia characteristics, such as forgetfulness and difficulties with concentration.

What Causes Progressive Supranuclear Palsy

A slow, progressive loss of brain cells in the area at the top of the brain stem is the general cause of PSP. Seldom is PSP an inherited condition, with this occurring in only one in one hundred cases. Interestingly, a gene factor oddity specific to PSP is seen in 95% of all reported cases.

Treatment

Parkinson's medications, such as those utilized as treatment for tremors and rigidity are often prescribed, but are generally not as effective in PSP. This is referred to as a drug resistant Parkinsonism. There is no known cure that will arrest the loss of brain cells as the disease progresses.

Corticobasal Ganglionic Degeneration

Introduction

So far, this chapter has focused on key symptoms of Parkinson's Plus diseases, and has provided examples of how they affect an individual physically and mentally. As I have throughout this book, I write from the perspective of a patient. Because I, too, suffer with Parkinson's Plus, I am able to convey the way this experience changes a life and puts your existence in a completely different perspective. I seek and read as much information as I am able regarding Parkinson's Plus conditions, and I put my background as an educational leader into the presentation of this information.

By way of a quick review, I remind you that there are the Multiple Systems Atrophies, which include Olivopontocerebellar Atrophy, Shy Drager Syndrome, and Striato-Nigral Degeneration. Other Parkinson's Plus conditions include Progressive Supranuclear Palsy, covered in the last section in this chapter, Dementia with Lewy Bodies, and the next condition I will describe, Corticobasal Ganglionic Degeneration.

Hallmark Symptoms of Corticobasal Ganglionic Degeneration

Corticobasal Ganglionic Degeneration (CBGD) overlaps considerably with PSP, as both are considered taupathies, or having to do with a defect in the tau gene. Due to this similarity, I have chosen to review this disease subsequent to my coverage of PSP in the previous section. The overlap of CBGD with PSP includes similarities in symptoms such as eye difficulties that affect tracking a moving object and difficulty initiating normal eye movement. It is also similar to a disease known as Fronto-temporal Dementia, as there is a factor of dementia that occurs with CBGD.

Speech is affected (dysarthria), swallowing suffers, and patients face what is known as alien limb phenomena. This involves a single limb moving in spite of the patient, as in the form of simply levitating, or unwanted or unplanned movements that seem alien to the person to whom the arm is attached. I have personally experienced this in the form of my right hand flapping uncontrollably, as it rises above my shoulder.

Parkinson's-like conditions that appear include rigidity that will typically affect one side (unilateral), occurring 79% of the time. Bradykinesia, also commonly found in Parkinson's Disease, manifests itself in CBGD as slow movements and is reported 71% of the time. Postural instability and walking gait difficulties are found in 45% of the cases. Dystonia, which is a common and often painful condition, causes the arm or hand to curl or assume a strange or awkward posture (43%). Tremors do occur with CBGD, but they are found as a result of movement, as opposed to the resting tremor of Parkinson's Disease. These are known as "action tremors." Myoclonic jerks will also appear, and these jerks may be tied to unexpected stimulus.

Cognitive issues, formerly considered less common in CBGD, have been recognized as a prominent feature of the illness. This takes the form of dementia and may be a major indicator of advanced disease. Patients frequently do not speak (aphasia), which eventually occurs in better than 50% of reported cases. Depression, common to all Parkinson's Plus Diseases, is generally a predictable issue. Bizarre behavioral signs, a lack of social

interest, and apathetic feelings, are all included in the psycho-
logical-emotional-behavioral issues that fit the profile of a CBGD
patient.

This disease is characterized by an asymmetric (PSP is symmetrical in its presentation, conversely), Levodopa-resistant, aki-
netic-rigid syndrome, with cortical features. The term "cortical
features" indicates that the disease affects the Cerebral Cortex, which presents in the form of dementia characteristics. So,
Cortico (meaning "of the cortex") -Basal Ganglionic (defined as
a disease of the movement center of the brain that is also involved in PD and other PD-like movement disorders) is a disease
that has a serious impact, causing both *movement difficulties*
and *dementia*. This disease begins in the patient's 50's or 60's,
and has an average survival of 8 years. There are many variables,
therefore there is no hard and fast rule regarding this prognosis.

Treatment

Levodopa and other prescription drugs used to treat Parkinsonism features such as rigidity or slowed movements, will often be
administered. It is important to add that CBGD, as well as other
Parkinson's Plus conditions, do not respond as effectively to this
dopamine replacement therapy. Other treatments would include drugs that focus on depression or other conditions found
in CBGD. There is no specific treatment that cures CBGD. It is
progressive and the best medical approach is to address specific
symptoms caused by the neuro-degeneration that occur with
this disease.

My Own Condition

For me personally, there are many similarities between the conditions described above and what I am currently experiencing, to one degree or another. I seem to have a number of the

CBGD issues, but certainly not all of them. A major difference you would find in my case relates to the concept of asymmetrical rigidity, stiffness and bradykinesia. Since the onset of my case, I have had *symmetrical* issues, with bilateral tremors, stiffness and coordination problems affecting both sides of my body equally (these occur unilaterally in CBGD and *also in typical* PD). This symmetry of Parkinsonian symptoms is consistent with PSP and some of the other Parkinson's Plus conditions. Although this doesn't rule out CBGD in my case (I am not attempting to diagnose my own case—I have an outstanding neurologist), I thought it might be interesting to the reader to know of those subtle differences.

The next section, as I continue to write from a patient's perspective, will focus on Shy Drager Syndrome, identified as one of the Multiple Systems Atrophy diseases.

Multiple Systems Atrophy

Introduction

Parkinson's Plus is indeed a diagnosis of a Parkinson's-like disease, with the movement disorder features of Parkinson's, but included are other complications. If the individual has problems with movement disorder issues on both sides of the body equally, in conjunction with eye movement issues affecting up and down gaze of the eyes, and a tendency to fall early in the course of the illness, the patient has Progressive Supranuclear Palsy. Corticobasal Ganglionic Degeneration is similar to PSP, with more of a tremor typical to Parkinson's Disease and alien limb phenomenon. PSP and CBGD are both known as taupathies, as they are connected with a defective "tau" gene that affects brain tissue.

Another group of Parkinson's Plus conditions are known as Multiple Systems Atrophy and customarily have included: Striato-Nigral Degeneration, Olivopontocerebellar Atrophy and Shy

Drager Syndrome. In recent years, doctors have come to the conclusion that these share a common pathology, with autonomic symptoms as the common thread. The result is rather than three distinct illnesses, Shy Drager has been renamed as Multiple Systems Atrophy (MSA), of which there are two subtypes with the autonomic factors being the unifying medical concern. These have been renamed by medical experts, or given a more current synonym, with a letter symbol placed after the acronym for Multiple Systems Atrophy (MSA).

Three Sub-types

Striato-Nigral Degeneration is signified as MSA-P, with the "P" representing Parkinsonian in its symptomatic presentation. MSA-C, is Multiple Systems Atrophy with an emphasis on Cerebellar issues, or Olivopontocerebellar Atrophy. The Cerebellum is involved in overall balance and coordination, and in MSA-C, this area of the brain is affected severely. Both MSA-P and MSA-C are subgroups of MSA, or Shy Drager Syndrome, and in this disease the autonomic systems are severely affected, thus bladder, bowel, heart rate, blood pressure, with a PD-like condition initially, are the hallmarks of this subtype.

According to the website www.pspinformation.com, symptoms of MSA may include the following:

> "stiffness or rigidity; freezing or slowed movements; postural instability, loss of balance; incoordination; orthostatic hypotension, or loss of blood pressure when standing; postural instability; dizziness, lightheadedness, fainting; male impotence; urinary difficulties; constipation; speech and swallowing difficulties; blurred vision; other symptoms: depression, confusion, dementia, seborrheic dermatitis, breathing difficulties due to vocal cord paralysis."

From my personal perspective, confusion and/or dementia cannot be overlooked as very challenging aspects of these diseases. The caregiver, family member or close friend will see the balance issues, tremors, lack of coordination, speech difficulty and notice the complaints from the patient concerning the autonomic symptoms. However, the depression and confusion/cognitive issues are as challenging as any of the others listed. Issues of changes in personality, behavior, cognitive slowing or confusion and depression are as serious and should not be assumed to be minor because they are not physically observable. I can't emphasize enough how some of these aspects have been very difficult for me and quite disheartening. Like any of the symptoms, these cognitive effects will increase and decrease in intensity, but this does not mean that they are not important issues. Because these diseases are affected by the fluctuations of brain transmitters and/or chemistry, the cognitive/emotional factors will ebb and flow, as well. Most Parkinson's Disease and Parkinson's Plus patients will experience these cognitive/emotional effects to a greater or lesser degree.

With that background, I will go into more detail concerning each of these MSA subtypes. Refer to the E-Medicine article entitled "Multiple Systems Atrophy" for a more detailed explanation of these MSA distinctions. See the web address for the "EMEDICINE" site, listed at the end of this chapter.

Keep in mind, I am not a medical doctor, but a layperson hoping to provide a well-defined, down-to-earth explanation for these conditions. My interest is primarily motivated by my own diagnosis of Parkinson's Plus. I have been told it could be either PSP or MSA, among other possible options.

Shy Drager Syndrome (MSA)

Multiple Systems Atrophy (Shy Drager) may appear to be a more typical case of PD in the first few years of disease onset, but as it progresses extreme drops in blood pressure upon rising from a chair, difficulty with bowel and bladder control, exaggerated pulse rate fluctuations and sexual impotence are the hallmarks as the disease progresses. Johnny Cash was thought to have Parkinson's Disease initially, and it is believed to have eventually been diagnosed as a case of MSA.

Striato-Nigral Degeneration (MSA-P)

This subtype is difficult in the initial years to distinguish from Parkinson's Disease. Tremors, balance issues, rigidity, speech and swallowing are all eventually affected. It will be distinguished from idiopathic PD by its faster onset and poor response to Levodopa therapy. The autonomic issues will also become progressively worse as the disease progresses.

Olivopontocerebellar Atrophy (MSA-C)

This one is similar to PD, but in addition to balance, ataxia (including walking/gait issues) and speech are affected more severely. Difficulty with the overall coordination of bodily movements is the striking difference between this and the other subtype.

As I have pointed out in this book earlier, the differences between these conditions may be difficult to discern for an extended period, and in some cases throughout the life of the patient. It is an often reported occurrence that a patient is diagnosed with PSP and upon study of the brain organ after death, evidence is found to show that the patient actually suffered with MSA. The converse is also true. Fifteen percent of all cases of Parkinson's Disease will eventually have a more refined diagnosis, and in some cases this determination isn't made until after the individual passes away. The point is, these conditions are more similar than different.

In corresponding with a prominently known doctor in the field of movement disorders at an earlier point in my experience, he explained that these diseases don't come in neat little packages. He continued that a case such as mine could actually be a hybrid condition, i.e., Parkinson's Disease/Dystonia, or another example would be Parkinson's/Alzheimer's (these are examples generalized to the movement disorder field, not me specifically).

These diseases are named for an emphasis on particular symptoms. This does not mean that the patient will have no overlap of symptoms. Similarly, a large portion of all MSA cases eventually include some autonomic difficulties, such as erectile dysfunction, constipation and bladder control issues, when the patient has the specific subtype of MSA-P or MSA-C.

In addition to the three diseases I have written about in this three part series, Dementia with Lewy Bodies is often considered to be a Parkinson's Plus. This disease has an overwhelming degree of emphasis on dementia characteristics, along with Parkinsonism. Some medical references will include Alzheimer's Disease in this category, as AD can begin with what appear to be PD-like tremors and other typical PD issues. Lou Gehrig's Disease (Amyotrophic Lateral Sclerosis or ALS) is mentioned in the category of Parkinson's Plus in a number of medical references, as well. I do not plan to investigate these as additional topics, primarily because I am focusing on the diseases that are customarily referred to as Parkinson's Plus. The Parkinson's Plus syndromes I have written about are the conditions that bear enough similarity to Parkinson's Disease that they are a major focus of the purpose for which I started this writing project.

In conclusion, it is my hope that there is a greater understanding that we now share about what Parkinson's Plus means and why it is not a vague, little-understood name given to a mysterious illness. Parkinson's Plus is a specific diagnosis and will in time, as my excellent neurologist has said, blossom into a more specific medical definition. It is not just another name for Parkinson's Disease and it does not respond well, in most cases, to dopamine replacement therapy, thus distinguishing itself from idiopathic PD. Parkinson's Plus does not by any means indicate that the doctor does not know what to call the condition.

Links on Parkinson's Plus Conditions and their Characteristics

A Site in Support of the Caregiver
http://caregivinghelp.org/index.php

A Stellar Life (Blog by Friend with M.S.)
http://dj-astellarlife.blogspot.com/

Cure PSP - Info on PSP and CBD
http://www.psp.org/

Day by Day with a Movement Disorder
http://movementdisorder.dirtybutter.com/

Day by Day Adventures of the PD Warrior
http://thepdwarrior.com/blog/

Emedicine Site
http://www.emedicine.com/NEURO/topic671.htm

From the Lab Rat's Desk
http://labratsdesk.wordpress.com/

Huntington's Disease Society of America
http://www.hdsa.org/

Janet Edmunson – Author/Speaker
http://www.janetedmunson.com/

Life with Shaky
http://lifewithshaky.blogspot.com/

METAMORPHIS of BTRFLYNANA and MSA
http://mobmsa.blogspot.com/

More Progressive Supranuclear Palsy Information
http://www.pspinformation.com/

MSA Patient Education Baylor University
http://www.bcm.edu/neurology/patient_education/pdcmdc/
msa.html

MSA Support Group Listings and Info
http://www.shy-drager.org/

Multiple Systems Atrophy (MSA) FAQ - Excellent
http://www.shy-drager.org/msa_faq.htm

Neurodegeneration: What is it and where are we?
http://www.jci.org/cgi/content/full/111/1/3?ck=nck

Parkinson's Disease Blog Network Site
http://www.parkinsonsblognetwork.com/

Parkinson's "Plus" Syndromes
http://www.cmdg.org/Movement_/Parkinsons_Plus/parkin-
sons_plus.htm

Parkinson's Plus Movement Conditions Defined

http://cpmcnet.columbia.edu/dept/neurology/movdis/learn/
glossary.html

Parkinson's Research Foundation Q & A
http://www.parkinsonresearchfoundation.org/

Parkinsonism: Road to Diagnosis (Navigating the Medical System)
http://pdroadtodx.blogspot.com/

Patients Like Me
http://www.patientslikeme.com/

PD Caregiver Site Parkinson's Plus Info
http://www.pdcaregiver.org/ParkinsonsPlus.html

Progressive Supranuclear Palsy Info
http://www.neurosy.org/disease/psp/pspinfo.shtml

PSP - Causes, Symptoms and Treatment
http://www.healthnewsflash.com/conditions/progressive_su-
pranuclear_palsy.php

PSP Defined and Explained
http://www.dizziness-and-balance.com/disorders/central/
movement/psp.htm

PSP Recognition (Poems for those with PSP)
http://www.psprecognition.com/index.asp?WCI=index

Shake, Rattle and Roll
http://katekelsall.typepad.com/my_weblog?

Shaky's World
http://shaakysworld.blogspot.com/

Society for PSP
http://www.psp.org/

Sophie's Search for a Cure Site (MSA)
http://www.rainlightfilms.com/

We Move Education re: Movement Disorders
http://www.wemove.org/

Chapter Four

Living with Parkinson's Plus

N THIS CHAPTER I have adapted individual articles written for the "PD Plus Me" online blog for the purpose of this book. Each one is an individual topic, and stands alone as a complete concept within the chapter as a whole. This chapter will focus on specific issues that affect learning to understand and live with a Parkinson's Plus condition.

MRI Procedure Scheduled

One year before the writing of this book, I had a scheduled magnetic resonance imaging (commonly known as MRI) to determine if there were any new findings or indicators to support a refinement of the diagnosis. The issues being considered were, namely: Was my case looking more like Progressive Supranuclear Palsy (PSP) or another of the Parkinson's Plus conditions, such as Multiple Systems Atrophy or Corticobasal Ganglionic Degeneration? Since I had what were indications of eye hangups, or eye movement dysfunctions, there was a strong case to be made for PSP. I did not expect anything earth shattering to come from this diagnostic procedure, but I hoped that it might shed more light on my case.

In months leading up to this MRI, I had heard an expert on movement disorders state that the typical Parkinson's Disease case takes two years of examination and testing to determine the actual diagnosis. *Parkinson's Plus* syndromes are presumably that much more difficult to come to a conclusion about and it is understandable that the process may take years. As my excellent physician told me, "We will need time to see your condition blossom in order to determine which Parkinson's Plus condition it will be" (my paraphrase).

This process of understanding and adapting to Parkinson's Plus is a long journey, and requires patience on the part of the patient and his caregiver. I know that the critical aspects for me in facing these uncertainties were then, and are now, maintaining my strong faith in God, enjoying each day with my family and friends, and having a positive outlook regarding the future. During these days I received much support from my online friends in the Parkinson's and Parkinson's Plus community. I continue to this day to participate in these online support communities, my regional Parkinson's and Parkinson's Plus support groups and I have many contacts through the blog I write called "PD Plus Me," which was a vehicle in the writing of this book.

The Magnetic Resonance Imaging Experience

Generally, all Parkinsonism patients (those with Parkinson's Disease or Parkinson's Plus syndrome) will need to undergo a magnetic resonance imaging (commonly called an MRI). There are a number of different types of machines, with the traditional one involving the patient being moved into a tube-like structure. Another choice is the open MRI, which caters to patients like me, who experience claustrophobia, when placed in enclosed spaces. Initially, I was not sure how I would do with the enclosed variety of the MRI procedure, but was asked to undergo this method due to its diagnostic accuracy for brain imaging. The first of several of these tests was most difficult, but I was able to endure the "closed" version of the MRI, which for me was a major success! I wasn't too pleased at first with my medical clinic's new MRI machine, as the tube they wanted to put me in was smaller in diameter than those I had experienced previously for spinal conditions. When the technician put me in for a trial run, I didn't feel there was much room for my large body (I am six-foot-four and 250 pounds)! I asked to come back out and then waited a few minutes to prepare myself. I wanted to go through with the test, because my neurologist had explained that a brain study is much more beneficial when it is taken in a closed MRI versus the open type (all of my previous brain related MRI's had been in an open machine). I wanted the neurologist and I to have the advantage of the best possible images, so, I asked the technician to put me in and said, "Let's get it done." The mild anti-anxiety medication prescribed by my neurologist helped considerably.

The radiology technician fitted a "mask" over my face, and it included a mirror which worked like a periscope on a submarine, allowing me to see out of the tube, though laying on my back eight inches from the top of the inside of the tube. With Mozart playing in my ears on headphones, I was able to look at my lovely and compassionate wife who stood at my feet looking directly into my eyes in the mirror. Her face and reassuring expression gave me the hope and courage to overcome my difficulties with claustrophobia and I was successful in staying calm for the 45 minutes we needed to get the study completed, including the last series of pictures taken after a brief interlude to put the "glowing water" (an isotope solution) in my bloodstream.

The reality is that many of the Parkinsonian or Extrapyramidal Diseases are not visible in these tests. That is universally true, although there are at times, exceptions. Certainly, any obvious manifestations of brain tissue atrophy will be visible and provide beneficial information for the neurologist to determine any necessary additional treatment options.

PD Plus Conditions are more Similar than Different

As we await the MRI results and some blood work outcomes that we are looking toward, one point stands out as an area needing clarity. PSP, MSA, Shy Drager, and CBGD are all forms of Parkinson's Plus, that much I have explained on many occasions. What I haven't said is that the longer I deal with these subjects, the more apparent it becomes that these are not only difficult to distinguish from each other in the first few years, but they are difficult to separate in dramatic fashion for the duration of the illness, in many cases. In order to get right to the point, an autopsy of the brain itself will in many cases be the only absolute diagnosis. They share so many symptoms with each other, and for that matter, with Idiopathic Parkinson's Disease, that they are all treated with virtually the same medications, in varying combinations and portions, depending on the patient. A diagnosis of PSP or MSA is actually, "It looks like you are likely to have PSP," or "It appears that you might have Shy Drager Syndrome." Rarely, is a neurologist able to state emphatically, "You have PSP." By the end of the first year of neurological treatment, I was told it was most likely PSP, given the options of the various Parkinson's Plus or Extrapyramidal conditions.

Secondly, since the treatments are virtually the same, and particularly so in my case as I am taking substantial doses of what are drugs typically dispensed in a fairly advanced case of Parkinson's Disease, it is not actually of great benefit to "fix a label" on this or any other case of Parkinson's Plus. The reason for this is that it will not mean a great deal of difference in the resulting treatment plan. Again, the various Parkinsonian conditions I have listed above, although they have very important nuances from one another, i.e., eye movement difficulties in PSP or autonomic interference in Shy Drager, they each include movement disorder issues, such as: bradykinesia (slow movements), stiffness, rigidity, tremors, cognitive slowing, swallowing difficulties and speech troubles. All of these symptoms are treatable, not curable, with PD related drugs, such as the following examples: Levodopa, Artane, anti-depressants and Azilect (neuro-protective purpose).

This suggests for me that I not worry about an absolute definition of the condition I face, but rather realize that, although frustrating, this lack of definition doesn't make a real difference in the prognosis or treatments that are available to me. My neurologist is providing me with an excellent course of treatment to reduce the negative effects of these various resulting physical and mental maladies, and that is really what is important!

Another issue I want to bring to your awareness regards the various movements that come with these conditions and their unique characteristics when compared to each other. There are tremors associated with these conditions, and particularly Parkinson's Disease, but in addition there are a number of other movement issues, including slowness (bradykinesia), unwanted and random movements (dyskinesia) and several others including Chorea and akinesia. I would encourage you to take the time to visit some of the excellent websites that I listed at the end of the previous chapter. These websites will give you a clear explanation of all of the associated movement problems and help to define these physical manifestations you may witness in your friend, loved one or spouse.

Answering the "Why Me?" Questions of Life

On Easter Sunday, of 2006, I posted an article on my PD Plus Me blog in which I asked the question "Why me?" regarding the diagnosis that happens to be mine.

Do you ever ask yourself, "Why me?" I have, and I do. I think that as Christians we know we are in God's hands, and yet we may have to wonder if our prayers are answered, at times.

I was interested in a discussion and sought no trite answers. Many individuals know and love personal favorite verses from the Bible, for example, which state things, such as, "God makes all things work together for good, for those who love Him" (my paraphrase of Romans 8:28). I am asking you as a human being, and each of you from a variety of faith or non-faith backgrounds, how you deal with the idea of good people having bad experiences or a bad turn, such as a serious medical condition.

A friend of mine said at the time, "Why not you, Dan? You are the believer and you are the one God knows can handle this." I know that comments such as these are intended as encouragement, but at times they seem incongruous with the actual circumstance I am facing.

I had worked through this in the first year following my diagnosis (2006) and had finally moved past the shock. I have dealt with this subject, then and now, and I find peace through my faith, although I am not going to say that I won't at times have doubts and questions. I have accepted the reality of the situation and have determined that it is time for me to live this thing out, with the same hope and realization of God's presence that I have relied on throughout my life when facing adversity.

Medications are Misunderstood as Cures

Last year Karrie and I went to our monthly Parkinson's Support Group meeting. At these meetings, the agenda generally involves having speakers present relevant information, or providing an opportunity to share ideas and experiences with one another as we deal with, for most participants, Parkinson's Disease. For a few of us, the challenge is a Parkinson's Plus condition of one type or another. One of the gentlemen in the group brought up an interesting and important point in this particular meeting that should be included in this book. He explained that he has come across a misconception that those without PD believe with regard to the medications taken for movement disorders, and their effects.

He explained that on a recent television program a character was accused of a crime. The accused happened to be an individual with Parkinson's Disease. In the process of defending this character, the attorney explained to the court that the gentleman being tried for a serious crime, was, in fact, a Parkinson's patient. The defendant's attorney explained that his client's PD condition should be understood as an extenuating circumstance when looking at the facts of the case. The prosecutor responded immediately that "the defendant could take medication and, when it took effect, be able to be a normal person." My support group friend wanted to make a point about this assumption and I wanted it to be included here, in this book.

My friend explained that this idea—that Parkinson's Disease sufferers merely need to take pills and they will be normal and have no ill effects from the disease—was a complete distortion. He was concerned that people generally believe this and it dawned on me that it would be important to explain this perspective.

In fact, as my friend explained, taking the various medicines that are prescribed, *designed primarily to address movement abnormalities*, does not make a patient completely *normal*. This belief is far from true and is problematic when those around the Parkinson's patient adhere to this perception.

Why is this an issue? My friend was trying to say that there is so much more to treating the medical issues caused by Parkinson's Disease (or other Parkinsonism disorders) than stopping unwanted movements, unfreezing of limbs, or the removal of a masked facial expression.

The truth is that every case is different, and *all patients experience a variety of additional symptoms in various combinations and degrees of severity.* First of all, remember that Parkinson's and other related Parkinsonian conditions, are not curable and involve a steady, progressive degeneration of nerve cells within the brain. As the brain cells fail and stop functioning, the physical problems worsen. In addition, various thinking-related or cognitive function issues begin to set in, also in varying degrees. Secondly, the medications do not address all of the resulting conditions that are brought on by the loss of these cells.

The goal of the medicines given to PD patients is to treat symptoms, such as: freezing, slowness of movement (bradykinesia), facial masking, drooling, reduction (not elimination) of tremors, and improvement of rigidity or stiffness. The various pills designed to accomplish these benefits do not bring an automatic success and have varying degrees of effectiveness, depending on the condition, its severity, and the number of years since the initial diagnosis. These drugs gradually lose their effectiveness as the average Parkinson's patient progressively loses his or her mobility. Subsequently, the patient will have more and more difficulty moving his/her mouth, hands, arms, legs and feet. Speech is gradually impacted more and more, as is the swallowing mechanism and other bodily functions and systems.

The point is that individuals who have these movement disorders are facing a decline, at varying rates. There is no cure, whether the treatment is brain surgery or medication, these approaches are not a panacea. Certainly these attempts are helpful to a point, but do not represent miracle cures. Your friend or family member facing PD or a PD Plus condition, is not "fine as long as they take their pills" as this show and others in the media have suggested (*can anyone forget the Rush Limbaugh rant accusing Michael J. Fox of not taking medication and thus faking his condition for sympathy?*) Medications help some more than others, but they do not cease all of the various symptoms or medical issues caused by these neurodegenerative conditions.

I want you to know that your loved ones are facing something much more insidious than this assumption would indicate. There are things going on all the time—cognitively, emotionally, and physically—that are not easily helped by any particular pill or surgery. These treatments are a great benefit and improve quality of life for most, but they do not fix the far reaching effects of PD and other similar movement disorders. None of us facing these illnesses would want to be without our medications, not even for a day! This does not mean that Parkinson's or Parkinson's Plus patients are "fine as long as we take our pills."

Parkinson's Disease: More Than Meets the Eye

There was an announcement in the local newspaper in the past year regarding Michael J. Fox that reminded me of a great confusion that exists regarding Parkinson's Disease and the extent of the symptoms involved. The announcement concerned a new FX television series coming out in the spring of 2009 that Michael J. Fox will be in as a wheelchair-bound character. His part will run for four episodes, and I look forward to watching, as I always appreciate seeing my hero acting in a current series. After explaining Mr. Fox's involvement in this television program, the article went on to give a quick review of how Parkinson's Disease is defined. How many times have I mentioned that Parkinson's is not just about unwanted movements?

The press indicated that Michael J. Fox works hard to control his undesired movements, which include tremors and rocking. It also stated that Parkinson's is a disease that causes undesirable movements that interfere with living. This is so far from being a complete explanation that it reminded me of how easily people become confused around those of us who have such a diagnosis. This includes those of us who have atypical Parkinsonism, which shares many of the same symptoms as Parkinson's Disease.

The emphasis seems to always be placed on how the individual looks. Here is the problem with basing your awareness of the suffering of a patient by looking for outward signs of tremors or dyskinesia. Parkinson's includes four major areas of movement issues:

Tremor - Typically a resting tremor, but does not occur in 30% of all patients

Rigidity - Patient has a general muscle stiffness that causes cogwheel jerking movements when asked to move a limb

Slowness - (Also known as bradykinesia) The body is forced to move slowly and in a restricted manner. It feels like you are walking waist deep in water and have to fight the force of the water against your body as it moves.

Postural Instability - The patient has trouble standing, walking with balance and eventually will begin to fall.

These four major symptom areas are generally focused on the physical aspects of the disease. Parkinson's and atypical Parkinson's disorders are caused by the deterioration of brain cells. Depending on the disease, these stem from a variety of factors. Parkinson's has brain degeneration in the Basal Ganglia, which leads to the above four major movement difficulties. In addition, other areas of the brain are damaged in varying degrees, causing slowed cognition, depression, anxiety, eye movement difficulties, swallowing and speech disturbances, fine motor coordination, freezing in place, insomnia, loss of smell, masked facial expression, skin problems, digestive difficulty, urinary problems, pain and stiffness of joints, and other specific problems too numerous to list. Generally, Parkinson's Plus syndromes include most of the same symptoms listed above due to degeneration of brain cells in the same areas as the PD patient. Additional neurological structures are affected in Parkinson's Plus diseases, thus they will have additional disabling factors.

So much is going on in the life of a Parkinson's or Parkinson's Plus patient, that it is doing a disservice to the patients and the medical profession to limit the public explanation of these diseases as being "undesired movements and tremors." *This description lends itself to the belief that this is a disease about embarrassment, rather than disability and suffering.* Taking medications to aid the Parkinson's patient is not just about reducing tremor and dyskinesia, thus improving the self esteem of the patient. Some of the above listed symptoms are improved with the various treatments available, but others are not affected, enough, or at all.

Parkinson's patients will tell you that embarrassment is not an important issue in the spectrum of issues they face. The internal, mental aspects are as difficult as a number of other issues, but they are not visible to others. When you are with your friend or loved one who has Parkinson's, please understand that they may not be moving as slowly or trembling as much, but inwardly they could be experiencing confusion or depression. In addition, there may be great fatigue, pain in the back or limbs, severe headache, nausea or weakness. Take it from me—there is a lot going on inwardly, that is rarely mentioned in a social circumstance.

Parkinson's is little understood in the general public and the media shares much of the blame for always putting the focus on "embarrassing movements" rather than the effects on the brain that cause great disability, gradually worse over time.

In the Parkinson's Disease community, publicity that is generated by such a special individual as Michael J. Fox, is of great benefit to the public. It is vitally important that we raise awareness about Parkinson's and other atypical Parkinsonism diseases. However, keep in mind the limited view of how these diseases are defined and let's all work to share the complete picture with interested people.

To Be Honest...

I have to be honest. Having Parkinson's Plus, Extrapyramidal Disorder, Abnormal Involuntary Movement Disorder, Progressive Supranuclear Palsy or whatever the medical profession chooses to call it, is apt to bring on a bought with depression, if not serious disillusionment. Let's not candy-coat it—I was, in the early months of the onset of my disease, and remain to this day, really disappointed. I look around and I see a beautiful family—a wonderful wife, three amazing sons and a very special daughter-in-law. My parents, brothers and sister, and extended family are the best. I have a church that is filled with supportive and caring friends that care, encourage us and pray for us regularly. I have the best friends on the face of the earth, and some that will pick me up and take me fishing or out for coffee. My home is just right for the four of us and our Black Lab, Jamie and 11 year old cat, Chester. I have my guitars, my books, my picturesque backyard and reasonable financial security (Author's note: this is not to say that the medical insurance situation is adequate in this country, at this time. Being disabled and losing my ability to work meant that four of us had to find other ways to get medical insurance coverage. There is no promise of the future in covering my family members. I am grateful to have the Medicare system, and am a huge advocate of this and other Social Security entitlements). So what eats at me?

I don't know if it sounds like I want too much, but I would like to have the prospects of a long life ahead. I want to remain mobile, and able to speak, see and feed myself. I want to be there for all three of my sons weddings (the first one was beautiful!), watch my grandchildren grow up, be able to take long walks (on foot, not scooter), turn gray with Karrie and finish the dreams I have planned involving using my doctorate to teach as a part time university professor in graduate school. I miss driving, which by default includes the selection of the next car—picking out the color, the interior, and making trivial decisions like the CD-player type or cloth versus leather interior. I regret that I will never find that little silly fishing boat I always planned on. All I ask for is a simple, aluminum craft with a five-horse power electric motor that I can put on a trailer and strap to the back of a worn, but clean, used Toyota pick-up. The sheer freedom as I would head off in the morning to fish for trout at Lake Perris, with man's best friend at my side riding shotgun, would have been a priceless joy.

I know. Face reality. It can't be that bad. Be thankful for what you have. Or how about, "None of us really have any promise of tomorrow," or, as someone recently quipped, "We all have our crosses to bear." With all sincerity, Jesus bore my cross and carried it all the way up Calvary's hill for me, so I wouldn't have to pay the price for my own sins.

Closing Prayer: Lord, I am listening. Speak to my heart. I promise to have an open mind and heart to hear what you want to teach me today about the situation in which I find myself. I just have to be honest. I need you to help me understand. –Amen

Gene Therapy

The following report was posted on a message board I belong to for those with Parkinson's Plus conditions.

"A clinical trial in 12 Parkinson's patients, reported today in 'The Lancet,' showed that direct insertion of foreign DNA into brain cells could safely reduce symptoms of the disease, in what is the first time gene therapy has been used successfully to treat a neuro-degenerative disease."– http://www.thelancet.com

The Parkinson's Plus conditions include a number of typical Parkinson's Disease conditions in a more severe form, are faster progressing, and result from the destruction of more areas of the brain than found in idiopathic PD (typical Parkinson's). These syndromes are: Multiple Systems Atrophy, Progressive Supranuclear Palsy, Corticobasal Ganglionic Degeneration, Striato-Nigral Degeneration, Olivopontocerebellar Atrophy, Shy Drager Syndrome and Dementia with Lewy Bodies. I have several links listed at the end of chapter three, where you can read in detail about the distinctions between the PD Plus syndromes and PD.

As I have said before, PD is a serious and progressive illness. It typically progresses more gradually than Parkinson's Plus disorders and the patient will tend to live a much longer life than those facing Parkinson's Plus. It can generally be said that Parkinson's Plus affects more areas of the brain in a more pronounced manner, while in PD the effect is primarily focused in the Basal Ganglia, which is the neurological center of physical movements. Doctors will say, however, that other areas of the brain are also harmed as a result of PD, but this effect is not as severe as in Parkinson's Plus.

I certainly have great empathy for my friends with Parkinson's Disease, and because of the aspects that are similar, I participate in Parkinson's Support Groups. The important thing to note here is that the differences are numerous and I wanted to point that out for clarity as we hear and read reports of treatments for Parkinson's Disease. Generalizing these to Parkinson's Plus Syndromes isn't possible, although any-thing that may treat the effects of neuro-degeneration brings hope that there may be a treatment that will help alleviate symptoms at some point. Remember, a treatment is not a cure.

I spoke with my wife, and my partner in fighting this illness, about a way to clarify the differences in a succinct manner and she responded with this paragraph that I can in no way im-prove upon:

> "That is great news about the gene therapy for PD. The folks with the classic form of PD will, hopefully, benefit from this! Making treatments affordable and available to the common person is likely the next hurdle with it but we can continue to be hopeful. As you know, Dan's assumed condition, Progressive Supranuclear Palsy (AKA "Parkinson's Plus") is somewhere outside the "Parkinson's" box on most of these advancements. Too few patients with PSP and other Parkinson's Plus Syndromes show good results from the Parkinson's treatments. But hope and a positive attitude are a must for all facing neuro-degenerative dis-eases!" – Karrie Brooks

I hope this helps to bring clarity to the question of how prog-ress made in fighting PD symptoms does or does not benefit Parkinson's Plus research, and that reminds us of the distinc-tions between the Plus Syndromes and Idiopathic PD. This sense of reality regarding the severity of Parkinson's Plus in no way should be taken as my resigning myself to any particular out-come or a sign of our taking a negative posture regarding my prognosis for the future. I place my hope in a God who loves each of us and has a perfect time and will for our lives. I know that He will see us through these struggles and allow us to face them with grace.

Living On with PD Plus

In 2007, my entire family and I enjoyed a camping trip to the local Palomar Mountain State Park, a place we have gone with our sons for the last 22 years, each and every summer, with the exception of just two years. I had a great opportunity to celebrate Father's Day in this way and it was so rewarding to catch 20 trout between my son, Mark, and I, and to be able to watch our adult children enjoying their time with each other as such close friends. We are blessed people to have children who have grown up to be such fine individuals. I am so proud of each of them. My scooter turned out to be a real blessing because I was able to tour the camp ground and also use it to take the quarter mile jaunt to Doane Pond. The fish were jumping!

The Riverside Parkinson's Support Group met today and continues to be a source of friendship, as well as an opportunity to learn about different treatments and approaches that benefit other members. We are continually inspired by the brave individuals who are both PD patients, as well as caregiver spouses. I am so thankful for our group and the friends we have grown to care for as we have participated.

I have an update on the hummingbird nest I told you about in the "God is Our Refuge" story (see chapter entitled, "With Faith I Will Go On"). The mother continues to faithfully shelter, protect, and yes, SAVE, what now appears to be just one baby hummingbird. It is so exciting because this past week the baby bird is showing its face and moving its gray wings a bit. The mother continues to sit on the nest and goes out foraging for nourishment and with great zeal returns to provide the sustenance that this tiny creature needs. Interestingly, this youngster does not have to ask. This small teacup of a nest continues to hang precariously and yet, somehow, safely from a thin, virtual twig of a limb and endures a daily strong afternoon breeze. God saves, shelters, comforts and provides for us in this same way. I am glad to have this visual reminder.

We are coming to a place of acceptance with the indicators we found on the MRI recently, as the Neurologist informed us that they had significance and confirmed further Parkinson's' Plus, and not idiopathic Parkinson's Disease. Each and every day is a blessing and a gift. I have the greatest partner and encourager in my lovely wife, who gives and gives of herself, patiently, in spite of her circumstances.

Acceptance Follows Grieving

As I review the things that I have been experiencing in the disease progression, I have been a bit surprised by my reaction to these changes. When will it let up and find a set point where I am able to just accept the situation as it is and move on? This is not reality—that I would expect such a case in my situation. The truth about it is that my disease is by nature a progressive and degenerative disorder. I can expect to have some ability lost to one degree or another generally on an ongoing basis. Little changes in my thinking, planning, language usage, balance, facial expression, eye movements (or lack thereof), weakness or numbness in my hands, and atrophy in my wrists and forearms—these are just a few examples. If I could step away from myself for three months at a time, I would see a fairly blatant difference in my balance, walking or an increased lack of blinking due to a time lapse such as a three-month stretch would bring.

Explaining these constant changes or losses to a close friend is hard, so much is internal and I am learning more and more that Parkinson's Plus, most likely the PSP variant, is something that can certainly be observed as outward manifestations are plentiful. However, I can't emphasize enough for my friends and family that the issues that are involved, symptomatically, go far beyond what can be viewed by another person. Much of what I face is very silent and internal, whether it be my body tremor, located primarily in my torso and affects my head, arms and legs almost constantly, or the mood disorder that appears nearly every day. In addition, I have slowed cognition and difficulty remembering obvious occurrences that have taken place in the last hour. My wife views the cognitive features of my condition as significant, and these signs cannot be minimized as so called "senior moments."

The good news is that I am able to find a great deal of information to help me track what these changes mean. I am so fortunate to have three message boards or on-line support groups that I belong to that really help: one for PSP, another for Shy-Drager, and a third for MSA. All of these groups overlap, believe it or not, and most of the people seem to be in a similar boat with me—there is an intersection between these various illnesses, all under the umbrella of Parkinson's Plus. Each case is different and the complexities make the diagnosis of the exact variant very problematic. Johnny Cash had Shy-Drager because his case focused on involuntary functions such as digestive, bladder, blood pressure variances and heart rate. Dudley Moore was afflicted with Progressive Supranuclear Palsy as his condition focused more on balance, speech, swallowing troubles, rigidity of the spine and neck, and eye movement problems. Others, such as Millie Kondracke, the main character in the made for TV movie called "Saving Milly," have severe tremors, speech disturbance and walking difficulty, and these symptoms resulted in the label, "Multiple Systems Atrophy." While participating in these on-line groups, I am able to share and receive a great education, much camaraderie, and understanding from those facing similar struggles. The members of these online communities are either individuals with the neurological illness, or family members who are care providers for someone else afflicted.

Understanding all of these things myself is one challenge; the other is helping those who love me and care about my circumstances to grasp the depth of the problems that are just not as apparent or visible. I know they believe me when I share with them, and that really helps!

I feel for my sons, Daniel, Mark, and Stephen, my daughter in-law, Jenny, and my wife, Karrie, for they have to deal with the concern and questions that affect them. I wish I could lift that burden more than anything in life! I know my parents and close family and friends struggle with the "Why?" question, too. I am so thankful for those who care so much, but I wish they didn't have to deal with these things.

I press on, knowing that each day is precious and there is a special new opportunity to make a difference in someone's life tomorrow.

Forced to Retire: The Effect of Parkinson's Plus on Career

Approximately two years before I completed this book, I had a wonderful opportunity to be recognized by a professional organization for my career accomplishments. This was also an opportunity to reflect on my life in public education that I will always treasure, and I find I miss considerably.

In 2007, my immediate family, friends and colleagues accompanied me as I attended an end of year awards banquet. I was invited in order to receive a special award from the professional organization I have belonged to for 19 years, an association of school administrators in our state. This organization has regional groups that each encompass a large area, which in most cases, consists of a county. Our group includes the school districts in our county, which number 23 school systems. Most of the assistant principals, principals, district managers and district level school administrators belong to this organization.

Each year our region hosts a recognition event such as this one and invites recipients to attend with their significant family members to walk across the stage for a moment of appreciation or special acknowledgment. I was blessed to be chosen to receive the "Memorial Leadership Award" which is given to an individual whose work exemplifies the standards a dearly departed colleague, for whom the award is named, demonstrated in his work as a school and district leader. It was a great honor to be in his shadow and I was thrilled, but humbled to be chosen to receive such a special recognition.

I appreciated so much the efforts of all who took part in recognizing me and those who were there in support from my wonderful district where I concluded my career. Also, there were a number of friends who were there from other districts in the region that I spent many years in as a principal and assistant superintendent of personnel. Seeing each of these people meant so much and touched me so deeply. My sons, my mother, my daughter-in-law and of course, my wife Karrie being present, and once again, supporting me, are to be thanked. Having my family there at this important occasion was so special. I also appreciated my close friends and colleagues who had been there for me throughout the two-year period in which Parkinson's Plus grew worse and forced me to retire.

Looking back over a 30-year period in which I worked in the public schools as an instructional aide, a teacher, a program coordinator, an assistant principal, principal, director and finally an assistant superintendent, I have nothing but joy and thanksgiving for the opportunity and privilege I had to teach and guide students and lead adults. I have been blessed with a long career that brought special meaning to my life and gave me many beautiful memories. It is only fitting that my oldest son,

Daniel, now carries on as a classroom teacher in upper elementary grades, which is where I started so many years ago. I am so proud that he chose such an important and vital career that invests in the lives of students. No one could be more suited to do this work, with his being so well read, possessing a warm personality and given his natural verbal skills.

Being disabled and consequently retired, is a hard pill to swallow, but knowing I did my best and was able to have the chance to make a difference, is something for which to be truly thankful.

I will always be grateful to all my fellow administrators and colleagues, along with my family and friends that were present at the awards event, for giving me this glimpse of the purpose and meaning that motivated me to get up and go to work, every day. I had a saying when I was working in public education: "I am going to *life*, not to *work*." This was because being a teacher of children and adults was my life's work and certainly one of the purposes for which God had me on this earth. I look forward to realizing other new purposes and reasons He will use my life in the future, even in the face of Parkinsonism Plus. We will keep moving forward, each and every day. As of this writing, I am in the studio, part time, recording album number three and planning to publish this book, both pursuits that give me great purpose as I walk on in my life.

The results of the MRI discussed earlier in this chapter were able to substantiate my neurologist's diagnosis of an atypical Parkinson's Plus condition. These changes he found in my brain tissue were important markers and will continue to be watched as I move forward in my fight against this disease process.

Parkinson's Plus Complexities

Parkinson's Plus shares many common symptoms and attributes with Parkinson's Disease, and yet there are a number of significant differences. Parkinson's Plus conditions are similar to Parkinson's Disease because they are neuro-degenerative in nature, but affect a number of functions that also originate from a variety of brain dysfunctions.

Parkinson's Disease is largely a disease of the Basal Ganglia, and specifically the Substantia Nigra, which is the neurological center of physical movements. Parkinson's Plus conditions typically have a basal ganglionic involvement, but other areas such as the Cerebellum and the Brainstem may be affected, in addition. Both are types of movement disorders that stem from the degeneration of brain structures and result in malfunctions that affect movement, coordination, cognition, and balance.

The Parkinson's Plus conditions include Multiple Systems Atrophy, Progressive Supranuclear Palsy and Corticobasal Ganglionic Degeneration. At the end of chapter three of this book, I have included a list of internet links on which you may find information that will explain and define a variety of movement disorders. These websites explain the differences as well as similarities between these various conditions.

Where the Confusion Lies

Like many patients with Parkinson's Plus, my condition started out looking like a possible case of Parkinson's Disease, in part, because I had an obvious "resting tremor." To date, the specific "Plus" disease I have is yet to be determined. This is a subject of frustration, although most cases of Parkinson's take up to two years to be determined, and the diagnosis often takes longer for Parkinson's Plus conditions.

Reflecting on Progression and Diagnosis

Every two or three months, I will notice a number of symptomatic changes. In the first year after diagnosis I returned to

Dr. N every six months. Presently, this schedule has been ratcheted up to every three months. After the passage of time, my excellent doctor is able to see how my condition blossoms further. "Blossoming" is a strange expression for something that is neurodegenerative in nature, and yet speaks to the need for certain hallmarks or symptoms to be clarified in order to determine which form of Parkinson's Plus I may be diagnosed with at some point. It is not uncommon for a case to go several years without a more specific diagnosis of Progressive Supranuclear Palsy or Multiple Systems Atrophy (as examples) being identified as the exact category of illness. I have always had great confidence in my doctor and am appreciative of the care he has exhibited in not drawing too narrow or hasty a conclusion without an adequate amount of evidence. He has given me nearly every relevant test available to modern medicine.

My wife and I attend a local Parkinson's support group meeting in our community, which helps us deal with the progressive nature of the disease. At the time of this writing, our recent meeting included an interesting speaker and provided a good opportunity to interact with each other about medications that are benefiting different patients, in varying ways. Our group frequently follows up our once monthly Tuesday seminars with a Sunday afternoon potluck, which gives us a chance to share a meal and fellowship with one another. We are able to share experiences about how our individual conditions are worsening, stabilizing or even spiraling out of control. The nature of Parkinson's Disease or Parkinson's Plus is a gradually degenerating process, so it helps to have a place to air these concerns, fears or the effects of the depression caused by these illnesses.

I was then, and continue to be now, concerned about my eye movement difficulty which is slowly getting more severe, as well as my declining walking coordination. My facial masking—startled looking eyes and frozen frown expression shown on my mouth—cause me concern. It is difficult not to be able, particularly when meds are wearing off, to give non-verbal signals of recognition, being pleased or responding in approval. These things come from the subtlety of a glance, expression or various forms of smiling. I may appear angry, frightened or confused, when, in fact, none of those things are necessarily the case! As someone who always wore a smile, I find it difficult not to be able to give these cues to friends, acquaintances and family members. Please bear with those you love who struggle with these limitations on non-verbal communication.

These are the things that weigh heavily on the mind of the Parkinson's or Parkinson's Plus patient. Sometimes the best things for me to do are to enjoy a cup of coffee and a long talk with my wife. By continuing with the writing of the songs I work on (I have written five new songs in the three years since my symptoms began), by tuning in a Dodgers baseball or a Lakers basketball game, getting into my televised political discussions on C-SPAN or CNN, or reading one of the numerous books I am always working on completing, I am able to channel my energy in a positive way. Why not focus on the joy of each day and make the most of the good things we have in our lives?

I continue to believe I have been blessed and have much for which to be thankful, including the friends and family that cared enough to read my online blog, which led to the writing of this book. Those who have spent time visiting and supporting me in a variety of ways, are priceless and have provided great encouragement on the hardest days. Sometimes, refocusing your attention on the good things that can be found in life, in the now, is the best strategy. I will now tackle this topic in the next section.

The Blessings of Each New Day

Each day can be viewed as a special and priceless gift. Since mid-2005, I have been experiencing eventful days. Having reached the conclusion of my career, from the standpoint of being disabled and thus no longer able to work in the profession of my choice, I am able to see how many of my family's practical needs are being met. I am blessed to have a pension, and fortunate that God gave me the strength to work in public schools for 30 years as I stayed in the same system throughout that time. We are fortunate to have a reasonable degree of financial security, which causes me to be truly thankful. Having a support group in our local community that is comprised of friends and spouses that are completely supportive is a huge plus in facing the challenges with which we all struggle. As support group members, we have an understanding between us that gives us all the courage and hope to go forward with each day.

Notwithstanding the material blessings that we have as a family in the way of security—a home, a church, a community, an income—this neurodegenerative disease is taking a toll on my human existence, physically and mentally. I struggle to walk and stand due to poor balance. I am in overall decline gradually over time. I am noticing more changes in the way my hands are becoming more awkward in their posture as they want to curl or close when I am not using them actively. My hands close tightly in my lap when I am resting and tend toward a claw-like posture when my arms are at my sides while standing or walking. My arms too, often bend at the elbow and hang in an odd posture at my sides, with a reduced swinging of my arms and lack of normal coordination. I have cramps in my arches, wrists, forearms, my lower back and particularly in my neck. My hands frequently feel partially numb and weakened. The strength in my hands as a life-long guitar player, and an athlete earlier in my life, is seemingly slipping away. My neck tightens in a bent posture and causes pain. My eyes have difficulty moving to track words when I read and thus are often very sore in the eye muscles, requiring Tylenol on a frequent basis.

I have interruptions in my speaking rhythm and a reduction of voice volume. I move slowly and can only walk a half-block or so without losing my coordination and strength. I have difficulty remembering to say the right name or finding the right word to plug into a sentence when speaking. I become very down in mood, a by-product of the depression that accompanies my Extrapyramidal* disease, and the Abnormal Involuntary Movement Disorder with which I have been diagnosed. My head moves nearly on a continuous basis in a nodding motion, improving some for a couple of hours when I take the dopamine replacement known as Sinemet. My hands "roll" in a constant tremor when I am in a crowd, with or without medicine, or at home when my medicines are wearing off. My legs shake frequently when I am seated. And finally, at times I have difficulty remembering information from just a few minutes earlier, and yet still have a great memory of things I have stored in my mind for many years. I frequently swallow wrongly, and have to cough for 10–15 minutes following most of my meals.

I share these things not to gain your pity, but rather to give you a sense of what a day is like for those of us dealing with these neurodegenerative diseases, including: Parkinson's Disease, Parkinson's Plus (i.e., Progressive Supranuclear Palsy and Multiple Systems Atrophy), Dystonia (something most of those with Parkinson's have as a by-product), Lou Gehrig's Disease, and Huntington's Disease. I have not named all of those conditions that have similar effects, but a number of the prominent ones.

I know that the prognosis each of us faces is not good, as we are expecting to continue to decline, some slowly, some moderately and others will progress at a rapid pace. What can we do about this condition of life?

I have found something that all people need—to find the beauty and opportunity in each new day. Waking up and recognizing that you have a new day before you to live, to love, to discover, to learn, to improve and to enjoy being with those you love, is a gift. Living today and making the most of that day, is a skill that I have learned since I retired and no longer have the demanding and inspiring career as an educational leader to motivate me. I have to find my own motivation in each new and special day!

I appreciate the beautiful mountains and hills around my home in the region I have grown to love since we moved here in 1987. The trees that surround our neighborhood are colorful reminders of God's presence and the gift that creation is for each of us. My wife (who is my best friend), my awesome grown kids, my black lab, my cat, our close family friends, and even my old pal—my guitar—are important reminders of the wonderful life I have been given. These things we take for granted at times in our lives, become so much more real and special because of the struggles we face, physically and mentally.

Life is precious to all of us. Being chronically ill makes it clearer to an individual just how priceless living is. Each and everyone one of us have an opportunity each day to thank God for the morning and realize the good things He has put in our lives. I wanted to be frank in my description in order to share what I am facing, so that you would understand what your loved one in the same situation may have to deal with on a typical day. In this way, you might be as supportive as my family and friends have consistently been for me throughout this two-year struggle. In addition, I hope it gives you reason to take stock of your life and consider the good things that God has placed there for today. None of us are able to control the future, but we can say, "This is the day the Lord has made, let us rejoice and be glad in it" (Psalms 118:24, New International Version).

*The term "Extrapyramidal" refers to those parts of the motor system that are not directly "Pyramidal," that is not the Corticospinal Tracts (upper motor neurons). It always includes the Basal Ganglia and often is considered to include Cerebellar systems, thus Parkinson's and Parkinson's Plus are examples of Extrapyramidal Disease.

Tremors and Other Movement Problems

This article will address movement issues as they are found commonly in Parkinson's and Parkinson's Plus conditions. As I wrote earlier in this book, in the section entitled "Symptoms of Parkinson's and PD Plus," I explained, "There are a variety of tremor types, including intention tremor, postural tremor, but the typical and most prevalent type is known as resting tremor. This tremor is characterized by an involuntary, rhythmic movement of an affected limb (hand, foot, arm, chin, lip, or head) and occurs during a time of rest. The more still the patient becomes the more likely the resting tremor is to be produced, involuntarily. Approximately 30 percent of all Parkinson's patients do not have a tremor of any kind."

Unwanted Movements, Tremors and their Types

Let's look at tremor and other unwanted movement problems more closely, from my personal perspective as a patient. Individuals with movement disorders experience a variety of issues, depending on the person. Tremor is less prevalent in some conditions and more likely to occur in others. As stated above, even in the case of Parkinson's, some PD patients have no tremor at all. Of course, 70 percent of those with

Parkinson's do have tremor, and it is usually the first notice-able difficulty. In my case, although I had other symptoms for several years that my wife and I now strongly suspect were a part of my movement disorder condition that has since been labeled Parkinson's Plus, it was the head nodding tremor that became bothersome and noticeable in the summer of 2005, which motivated me to go and ask a doctor about what was going on.

Titubation

Head nodding tremor (also known as "titubation"*) is consid-ered much less common in Parkinson's Disease (although it is reported by a measurable number of patients, even in idiopathic Parkinson's) but is found in some Parkinson's Plus conditions, particularly Multiple Systems Atrophy, and in particular, Olivo-pontocerebellar Atrophy. As I have continually sought informa-tion concerning my case, more and more websites and articles have included tremors of the head and torso as conditions in-cluded with Parkinson's Disease, although I do not have typical Parkinson's Disease. However, head nodding is clearly indicated in some cases of Parkinson's Plus, such as Olivopontocerebellar Atrophy.

Resting Tremor

When my head nodding tremor became noticeable initially, it was something that was much more prominent during times of resting, typically when sitting and watching television, read-ing or listening to someone speak. I often would joke, "Don't assume I am agreeing with you when you are speaking with me, as it appears that I am nodding 'yes!'" This helps to lighten the situation up and gives friends and family a chance to take a breath and laugh with me.

After nearly three years since that original head nodding tremor sign was first noticed, I found that the tremors I deal with are not just of the resting variety. Although initially I had head tremors that appeared during rest, such as sitting watching TV or listening to someone speak while sharing a cup of coffee, as time went on I realized that I shake in my arms, legs, hands, feet and torso, much of the time. This includes when I am walking or standing. My right and/or left arm and hand shake when I am standing or walking, coupled with my fingers curling under in both hands on one side or the other. My right arm draws up at my side, giving it an awkward appearance. The tremor in my torso that I experience regularly, may be better described as a rhythmic, trembling sensation inside my chest.

Stress and Tremors

Tremors are aggravated by emotions, long periods of sitting and listening, or being in the presence of groups of people. My tremors are usually worst during a church service, watching a movie or during a conversation in which I am doing more listening than speaking. Tremors in Parkinson's result from a loss of dopamine cells located in the Basal Ganglia, which is the movement center of the brain. Tremors in Parkinson's Disease, and possibly other similar movement disorders, result from a loss of Basal Ganglia cells that were damaged by exposure to environmental toxins or some form of head trauma. Although patients rarely come to know what led to their condition, we all develop possible notions of what we think may have occurred. In 15 percent of the cases, these Parkinson's disorders result from some form of inheritable factor, or genetic link. Nonetheless, a loss of cells or neuro-degeneration, particularly in the Basal Ganglia, will be a certain cause of tremors.

Postural Tremor

In addition to resting tremors, it is my opinion I also experience what is best described as postural tremors. Postural tremors are another form of rhythmic shaking that result when a body part or extremity is held in a suspended position, such as a hand held out in front of you or dangled while resting an elbow on the lap. I shake when I am standing, walking or reaching for my wife to take her hand or put my arm around her shoulder. Each time I do this very natural movement, I will shake and thus begin to shake her. I have come to the place where I have to restrict my natural affectionate personality as I do not want to cause her to shake along with me. These displays of affection have to be brief, which means I may not put an arm around my wife for any length time while sitting in church or a theater. In addition, when I enter a room full of people, I will shake the most of any other time. It is more difficult for me to be with groups of people, although it is something I naturally enjoy as a part of my interests such as teaching, socializing or performing music.

Dyskinesia

Another movement symptom I encounter is known as "dyskinesia," which is an unwanted writhing or random dance-like movement of the arms, legs, hands or head. It is distinguishable from a resting or postural tremor in that its random, wild appearance is contrary to the rhythmic, patterned appearance that characterizes typical tremors found in Parkinson's or Parkinson's-like conditions. The reason dyskinesia occurs is that our medicines, such as Levodopa, are wearing off, and thus causing an additional, unwanted movement. Taking Levodopa is necessary due to the loss of Basal Ganglia cells in the movement center of the brain. By the time one begins to recognize tremors are beginning to occur, a movement disorder patient has more than likely lost approximately 70 percent of these dopamine cells.

Levodopa Treatment

Levodopa replaces dopamine, but only temporarily, as it has a limited time frame that it is effective (this is known as the "half life"). The time Levodopa works moderately well for me is approximately two-and-a-half hours. This half life varies from person to person. In my case as a Parkinson's Plus patient, Levodopa has much less effectiveness than it does for individuals with Parkinson's Disease, and this sign is one of several factors that serve as a basis for a Parkinson's Plus diagnosis.

Levodopa doesn't cure Parkinson's or Parkinson's Plus, but it provides temporary relief from tremors, stiffness or slow movements. It helps patients that freeze to be able to move again, or a PD patient would be stuck for an undetermined length of time. Thus, Levodopa is very necessary for the patient, but will result in moderate or severe dyskinesia. You may notice your loved one, friend or me not only shaking with tremors, but also exhibiting a more random and writhing type of movement. This is dyskinesia and is an unavoidable part of the vitally important Levodopa treatment. The "wearing off" of Levodopa results in dyskinesia in many patients that take this medicine. There is a trade-off, but most patients would consider the benefits to outweigh these side effects.

Many neurologists start patients on dopamine agonists, such as Mirapex or Requip, as an alternative to Levodopa. It is thought that these control unwanted movements and tremors, but are gentler on the patient in the early stages of PD. When these agonists are effective, the patient can avoid the side effects of Levodopa and postpone the need for its use until a later time in the illness.

Tremors and dyskinesia will cause unwanted movements. Additionally, the rigidity of Parkinson's or Parkinson's Plus, will cause a patient to have stiffness in the wrists, ankles, or neck, and present with a masked-like facial expression. The Parkinson's Plus conditions that will cause the patient to experience rigidity, include: Progressive Supranuclear Palsy, Olivopontocerebellar Atrophy, and Corticobasal Ganglionic Degeneration. This stiffness leads to difficulty rising from a chair, a difficulty in walking with any ease and causes severe soreness of joints and muscles. I am having a steadily progressing onset of rigidity in my condition, and thus my pain is also increasing over time.

Bradykinesia

Slowness of movement, or "bradykinesia," is a fourth symptom that should be included in this discussion, because it is another of the major factors that affect movements. Parkinson's medications such as Levodopa (brand name Sinemet) also may help the patient to overcome this slowness of movement, as it too stems from brain cell loss from one of these movement disorder conditions. This slowness is not to be confused with fatigue or weakness, but it is a specific restricting of movement resulting from a malfunction of neurotransmitters in the brain itself.

No one article in a periodical or section in a book can possibly include all of the information and detail that could be explored in such a topic. My goal in this section was to share with those who have friends or family members experiencing similar conditions, a bit more detail regarding tremors, dyskinesia, rigidity and bradykinesia.

Titubation - "a tremor of the head and sometimes trunk, commonly seen in Cerebellar disease" – http://medical-dictionary.thefreedictionary.com/titubation

Chorea Movements

During the course of this illness, I have experienced unwanted movements, called Chorea. These movements appear in the form of twisting, writhing, dance like movements of the wrists, hands, fingers, arms, and head. Such movements can be associated with a Parkinson's Plus syndrome, or Huntington's disease. My neurologist is treating these unwanted movements. In the process of receiving this treatment, there has been a period of adjustment. We have remained in close contact with our neurologist throughout this time.

In addition to concerns about Chorea movements, I have been facing trouble involving the use of my hands. I have had an increasing difficulty in feeling control and coordination over my hands and fingers. This has led to difficulty with typing, including keyboarding for this blog, and has also affected my guitar playing. Needless to say, this has caused much concern, and even some fear. Medically, there have been some adjustments which have resulted in a degree of improvement. Typing and guitar playing remain difficult but I have hope that these skills may return to full force. With regard to typing, this article is being written orally, through a microphone, using a voice-activated software program. This program was sent to us as a gift from one of our regular blog reader friends. What a wonderful gift!

My walking is slower and involves much shorter steps than in previous months. My facial masking has become more pronounced, as have my unpleasant eye movements. I'm adapting to these changes to the best of my ability. There is still much to be thankful for, with my family by my side, and my special wife, who is always there to assist and guide me.

Support Groups Make a Difference

Recently, my wife and I attended our support group that is based in a neighboring community that is very close to our own city. This was our third month in attendance, and it has proven to be a very beneficial, educational and supportive environment. The group consists of approximately 20 Parkinson's patients and a few individuals with Parkinson's Plus (including me) who come together each month. There are excellent, practical speakers that visit and make presentations. This month we had a pharmacist who specializes in Parkinson's drugs and the interactions to be aware of when taking drugs for a variety of conditions caused by Parkinson's Disease. We have medications that treat us for various conditions, including: tremors, joint and muscle stiffness, slow movements, depression, sleep disorders, and over-salivation, just to name a few. These drugs must be taken with a knowledge of their effectiveness, along with an awareness of their drug interaction issues and possible side effects. We were able to ask questions and were given some excellent information about various drug therapies and issues to watch for as we proceed in taking these prescribed medications as a part of our treatment plan.

The group consists of patients and their spouses, some single individuals and a volunteer group leader, who is enthusiastic and knowledgeable about a variety of Parkinson's subjects. My wife and I are benefiting, both from a learning standpoint, and also with regard to forging relationships with new friends who share the same struggles and challenges that we do each and every day. What a blessing to have such a group to attend and to know they understand and care!

Initially, we didn't know of such a group and were fortunate to attend one in a city an hour away from our home. We still stay in touch with this, our original support group, and attend their meetings as often as we are able. In January of 2006, we walked into our first support group and I remember realizing for the first time that we were with other people that were dealing with many of the same issues we were, i.e., careers interrupted, the effect on your children, the depression that results from the losses that are by-products of such a condition entering your life at a very inconvenient time and the desire to find out what can be done to treat such an illness. I found much comfort in a group of people that were so immediately understanding and encouraging in such a time of questions and disillusionment.

A year later, we found a similar group, but one that was near to home and has a family-close kind of feeling tone. We are going to be apart of this group for many years to come, and I thank God for the provision of a support group that provides both a learning opportunity, along with genuine fellowship and mutual concern.

Eye Movements/Blepharospasm

I face an ever increasing difficulty with my eyes moving in ways I do not appreciate (why won't they just cooperate?). In reality the eye movement troubles, which include my eyelids trying to close when I am listening to someone speak or riding in the car, are a product of brain dysfunction resulting from my neurological disorder. My eyes also tend to turn up in my eyelids, which causes some eye muscle pain. These symptoms do not persist, but are most noticeable when under stress or when I need to sit and listen for a long period of time.

Gait Difficulty

In addition, I have an increasingly difficult time with my walking gait. It is becoming less smooth and more like staggering, literally. In addition, when my medicines wear off, I will tend to shuffle with short steps.

Balance

Finally, twice in the recent weeks, I have fallen back into my chair when attempting to stand. The second of these two occurrences was accompanied by my nearly falling to the floor! My wife was right there and caught me before the chair I had been sitting on went one direction, while I would have spilled on the floor in the other. Thank God for my wonderful wife who was right there to grab my arm and steady me before I hit the floor. I must say that has not been a common occurrence in the past, but is a sobering reminder of the difficulties that this disease may hold for me in the future on a more regular basis. The answer, of course, is to be more proactive and rise with more care, making sure I have something to hold onto or a family member is nearby when I need to get up.

Friends and Family Make a Difference for the PD or PD Plus Patient

I am encouraged by a number things, including the many friends who remain in contact with me and give me their heartfelt support. I continue to marvel at the support of all our friends and family! My co-workers and leaders in the school district from which I have retired have shown so much kindness and caring. We have a church family too, which is unparalleled in the genuine care and love they show to our family. We are truly blessed!

Using a Mobility Scooter

We live in a great area, where there are mountain views, loads of greenbelts consisting of "woods", trails that go through all of these small forests, and a beautiful, paved walking path that encircles the entire planned community. The area is appropriately called "Hidden Springs" and has so much to offer to an individual with some measure of disability, which in my case, includes difficulty with mobility. Having a mobility scooter is a real blessing. The fact that it is Dodger blue, is no accident!

Let me explain the way I use this device and how I choose when and where to use such assistance devices. I have a cane; a beautifully carved cane given to me by some dear friends (you know who you are!). I use the cane around the house, at church, while visiting friends or if I go into a small store or restaurant. I have a wheelchair, provided by insurance, to go to larger stores, when I am assisted by my wife. My rule of thumb is to take the wheelchair when we go to a mid-sized to larger store when I will need to shop with my wife for a longer period of time.

The mobility scooter is useful when we take long walks in our scenic community, when we visit the mall, a large box store such as Costco, or if we have an outing that takes in a large area such as an amusement park or a walk around a town. It is important to note that a scooter lift is needed in order to make this system work. Ours is a hydraulic lift that locks the scooter in after raising it. We then are able to take it on the road, even if we are going camping!

These aids are needed because I have a balance and coordination problem that affects my ability to walk. It causes me to walk in an uncoordinated manner, such as my left foot turning in toward my right, and a stiff-man-style marching gait. In addition, my legs move slowly and get fatigued in 10 to 15 minutes.

I am thankful for the ability we had to purchase this scooter. Not everyone is as fortunate, and we know that this adds to our quality of life.

On Appreciating Caregivers

I must say that I have a great appreciation for what a caregiver goes through in the process of being the lifeline for a patient. I am a patient with a Parkinson's Plus syndrome, yet to be determined if it is definitely either MSA or PSP. I am only in the third year of my life with this disease, but I know that my behavior is affected. I see my wife dealing with the slow responses, the lack of facial expression or the frowning appearance that I unintentionally show. I "get" that I can be testy and, at times, it is due to medications that are changed or causing side effects. She goes through the times of depression, loss, fear, my frustration with the reactions of people, and the sadness that I can no longer work or drive. I marvel at how patient she is and the space she allows me in which to express my great disillusionment.

My very special wife has to help me get in and out of the car, and into the wheelchair, just to go to the movies or to shop in a store. I must say, my heart breaks more for her than it does me. I also realize that I am not as far along as some patients some of you care for, with whom you are facing greater challenges. I just want you to know, there is so much going on, inwardly, that we, as patients, have a hard time explaining.

I am more verbal than most, and I had the benefit of being a communicator by profession prior to the onset of this disease. However, it is considerably harder to get thoughts from the idea stage to the verbal output level. Writing, due to my typing proficiency, is by far the best form of communication for me now. This reminds me of a line in the Ringo Starr song, "You know it don't come easy...". When I can't type, and it has been very difficult for me at times, I have the availability of voice-activated software to keep me going.

I participate in forums where patients and caregivers post thoughts, concerns, questions, gripes and fears. These forums are vitally important as a source of support, encouragement and beneficial ideas that are needed in dealing with the lives in a family facing this challenge. Sometimes the things written are from the perspective of the caregiver and they reflect a great deal of frustration and disappointment about the behavior and or disabilities of the patient. It is painful to see in print sometimes how much pain we cause spouses and other family members. I know it is true. In reading postings found on message boards focused on Parkinson's Plus diseases, I sometimes get the feeling that it is inevitable that a Parkinson's Plus patient will become difficult, even rude and unkind. I refuse to believe that I could ever show anything but love and appreciation toward my wife, who is my best friend and my caregiver. I don't know where I would be without her.

From a patient perspective, sometimes it hurts to read about how we are perceived, notwithstanding the truth it represents. However, through these honestly expressed questions and concerns, I do learn much about what my wife and caregiver deals with, when I take time to listen to that perspective. I am fortunate to have someone who is there for me and truly cares. Not everyone in my situation can make that statement. So, I say, to all caregivers, "Thank you!" And, if I might add, please remember we are listening.

Dysarthria — Speech Difficulty

The American Speech-Language and Hearing Association's website defines dysarthria as,

"After a stroke or other brain injury, the muscles of the mouth, face, and respiratory system may become weak, move slowly, or not move at all. The resulting speech condition is called dysarthria. The type and severity of dysarthria depends on which area of the nervous system is affected." – Dysarthria(n.d.). Available from the Web site of the American Speech-Language-Hearing Association: http://www.asha.org/public/speech/disorders/dysarthria.htm. All Rights Reserved.

Among the causes of dysarthria are neuro-degenerative conditions such as Parkinson's or Parkinson's Plus. It is common for the individual to have difficulty with slurring speech, low volume of voice, slowness of speaking, and difficulty with moving the mouth, including the lips, jaw and tongue. Additionally, the rhythm of speech or cadence, coupled with monotone speech quality or tone may be added difficulties, according to these speech experts. Cognitive problems the PD or atypical parkinsonism patient also tends to struggle with, just make this whole communication problem more troubling.

Effect on Verbal Skills

In speaking with my wife recently, it occurred to me that one of the most difficult aspects of this movement disorder I am experiencing is the way it has affected my communication ability. Being a lifetime educator, including teaching and administration, makes this problem even more frustrating. I began to sing and entertain crowds at the age of 10, and I have been a performing musician, and primarily a singer/guitarist, all of my adult life. So when I tell you that I am struggling with my speech and it is affecting me emotionally, it is no small issue.

I find myself having difficulty trying to say "thank you" at retirement events or when I get on the phone to make a business call, i.e., making camping reservations, I struggle to express myself. This is maddening! I think what makes my difficulty with speech the most difficult, is when I am on the phone and the person I am talking to has no idea that when I struggle to speak quickly enough to answer questions or make requests, it is not me being unprepared or just plain "dense." It is humbling, to say the least, to hear the frustration on the other end of the phone when I come across as unprepared or less than sophisticated. If I am not careful, it might really hurt my pride!

I find that my words come out slowly and I have to pause to put the next phrase together. Or I may have trouble thinking of a word, forming a word with the right inflection, or speaking in an authoritative enough manner to be understood for my intended meaning. I seem to have a "one pitch fits all" voice quality, though I have spent my life professionally developing the knowledge and skill to speak in a variety of voice levels and styles, in order to move an audience, motivate my listener, give clear directions, or show deep emotions. When my medicines are working well, I have less trouble, but it doesn't ever simply go away. I seem to have this struggle at all times, but particularly with any kind of stress or pressure to make a point clear when needed.

This may take the form of ordering food or drink at a counter with people waiting in line behind me. I will have trouble saying, "a grande Cafe Latte, sugar free hazelnut, with no whipped cream, please." I may say, "Cafe Latte, uh, please, (long pause) uh hazel sugar, uh hazel sugar free, whipped please—is that right?" (pause—by this time the server is getting frustrated, but most are very patient and kind!) I continue, "No, I am not sure. I mean sugar free hazelnut." While this is happening, I feel a bit confused and I have a feeling in my lips and tongue that is as though they do not want to move in concert. The muscles in my mouth do not want to respond effectively or in a coordinated manner.

This example is a practical situation that actually occurs, regularly, especially since I am on disability-retirement, and have many more opportunities to go with my wife to Starbucks, a fact that I find appealing! Nevertheless, this is one of the most hurtful aspects of having an involuntary, abnormal movement disorder, such as that with which I have been diagnosed. I struggle with oral communication, something I once considered to be a strong-suit of mine. I prided myself on speaking well, and winning people through forthright, positive communication.

When you think of Parkinson's Disease or atypical Parkinson's disorders, such as Parkinson's Plus, you may primarily picture a person who shakes, has tremors and struggles to move at a normal speed when walking. There is so much more to these conditions, including the recent topic I discussed regarding swallowing. This swallowing issue is not too distant in relationship to the speech problem, or dysarthria, I am writing about tonight.

When you are with someone who has PD or PD Plus, it helps the patient for you to remember, they may speak slowly, or in a soft voice or they may have difficulty finding the right words, but this doesn't mean the individual is any less intelligent than they were before getting this disease. They are dealing with a speech difficulty caused by a condition that has affected the brain's ability to control movement, and the speech mechanism is part of the movement processes of the brain.

Experts, such as those at the American Speech-Language-Hearing Association (http://www.asha.org/default.htm), would be better equipped to tell you how it is that these mechanisms are affected, along with a neurologist or movement disorder specialist, who would explain the neurological aspects of this problem. I am speaking as a patient and a friend, and I want you to know, this symptom is one of the most frustrating and difficult to accept. It is a constant reminder that you are different and that you have lost abilities that you may have taken for granted, or in my case, counted on as a primary skill in a professional career. Communication was what I depended on as I led, taught and shared with fellow educators, students, parents, attorneys and administrators. Ironically, my area of concentration for my bachelor of arts degree at California State University, Long Beach, was Speech Communications.

I trust this information will be of benefit to you as you encounter those in your life that are struggling with a movement disorder that has, as a byproduct, caused dysarthria.

Retirement Recognition

Approximately two years before the completion of this book, I was blessed by my school district from which I retired to be recognized at a meeting and presented with a beautiful plaque and hand-made quilt. These gifts were so thoughtful and were a joy to receive. The thought that went into them was so very appreciated by my family and me. It was also a very touching and memorable evening for my sons, my daughter-in-law, my wife and me.

Retiring early due to this neurological disease was something I had to struggle with accepting, having loved my career and the opportunity it afforded me to work with students, teachers, staff, managers, board members and parents. What a wonderful opportunity—being able to make a difference in other's lives! I mentioned in another section that I used to say, "I'm going to life, not to work." Teaching and later being a principal and district administrator, was the perfect job for me. Leaving my career early, continues to be a reminder that this neuro-degenerative condition has taken a large toll.

The evening took place at a school board meeting and the district leadership was very gracious in the comments they made about my life's work. The showing of teachers, support staff, fellow mangers and administrators who took the time to be there, was so moving. As I looked around the room, at the standing room only crowd, I was moved to tears. As I spoke my words of thanks and concluding comments about the privilege and joy it was to be a public schools educator, many of us in the room were emotional. I know it was a hard night for my loving wife, Karrie, to sit and watch me get through this challenge. It was a challenge because of the emotions and the impact, true, but also due to my tremors, cognitive effects and balance problems derived from the Parkinson's Plus condition. I had to take my time and pause, as I choked back tears and reviewed a life fulfilled working with kids and leading/supervising adults.

I am a fortunate man. God opened the doors that led to my progress in my career and by His grace I was able to do some good with the partnership and help of many talented and dedicated people. It is hard to understand why I didn't get to continue, and yet each day I spend with my wife and family as an early retiree, I realize how much I missed in the years I was gone on average, 11 hours each day.

I want to express my thanks and appreciation to all those in my school district for their generous demonstration of love and respect. I was moved and humbled by this experience. I will miss you all, and remember the great three years I spent working with you as I put a cap on a beloved career.

HR-3 Stem Cell Research

We have found a new support group, located in our community and based at a local church. The group is not affiliated with the church, but it is a wonderful environment for meetings. Each month an expert comes and shares some information meant to assist and inform us as patients, or care givers. I am excited about the relationships we are building and the network of support for the future! There are some great people and it is not only helpful, but enjoyable to be with these friends, who share the struggle with PD or PD Plus in my case.

I have been following the stem cell legislation discussion going on in Congress, as I am sure many of you have as well. On January 11, the House of Representatives approved expanded federal funding for Stem Cell Research. The bill, HR 3, is called the Stem Cell Research Enhancement Act of 2007 (see New York Times, Kirkpatrick, January 12, 2007).

I find it interesting that the type of research being proposed was already signed into law by President George W. Bush a few years ago! He approved research on existing lines of embryonic stem cells, which were thought at the time to be approximately, 70-75 stem cell lines or groups. In reality, there were only approximately 21 available, and most of them were contaminated and not useful for stem cell research. The issue is: When a couple creates embryos in a fertility clinic they may use between three-five for implantation in the womb (as an example). If they created and froze 12-15 originally and have completed the purpose they intended for their development, they then determine to dispose of the remaining embryos. This is current practice and is legal, being done all over the country in privately funded clinics. The question isn't whether to legalize embryonic stem cell research; it is already legal! The question before the Senate and then President Bush to sign into law (or veto it as he did recently) is whether to expand the availability of embryonic stem cells by allowing parents who are in the process of disposing of the embryos (consisting of 8, 10 or maybe 16 cells, total), to have the option of donating this tissue for research use. This would then allow the research to grow to a reasonable size and hopefully bring about some medical breakthroughs that could save lives. Parkinson's, spinal cord injuries and diabetes are three of the conditions that may benefit.

There is a lot of discussion about other stem cells, including: adult, umbilical and the amniotic variety. Doctor's and scientists believe that we need to conduct research using all of the above! Why limit research to these three forms and not include embryonic, since: 1) President Bush made this research a legally funded process, while limiting the number of stem cells available, enough to cripple the process; 2) The vast majority of experts (scientists and doctors, not philosophers or politicians) have stated emphatically that the embryonic stem cells are by far the most effective.

Why are embryonic stem cells more effective? Because they are much more of a clean slate and have not developed any specificity, thus when implanted in brain tissue they are able to mimic those cells and begin to reproduce thereby creating (theoretically) new dopamine cells. These dopamine cells are being lost in the PD patient, thus the condition results. Adult cells are much narrower in their ability to adapt because they have already taken a specific form, thus they don't provide the degree of flexibility, which is the beauty of the embryonic stem cells.

I am not intending to persuade you, nor do I have anything but respect for those who would not support this research, if you are making your decision based on facts and a true knowledge of the issue. The problem is that the broader public does not know that this research is presently legal, but that the number of lines was limited. When the original legislation went through with this limitation, the President was attempting to compromise, appealing to the pro-life movement, while still promoting the research using embryonic stem cells. The parents are going to dispose of these cells unless they are allowed to donate them. Presently, they can legally donate them to research and research is legally conducted. The difference is that the federal government would be providing vitally needed funding for this research, therefore it could be expanded.

Please consider how this form of research, which would allow something with the power to save lives and is presently being disposed of every day, to be donated. If this donation process is allowed these embryonic cells would be giving life to PD patients and others who desperately need a cure for their diseases. Wasting this valuable resource by simply discarding these cells, is a waste of invaluable, life saving resources.

I hope my layman's explanation is helpful to you in providing information for your future discussions and determination of your viewpoint.

Embryonic Stem Cell Research

I read with interest a summary of a topic that President Bush referred to in his 2008 State of the Union speech.There were some thought provoking statements that he made, which included a reference to new discoveries regarding stem cell research making the use of embryonic stem cells obsolete. To quote a representative of the Family Research Council's summary of this reference:

> *"A high mark came when the President explained how advances in science have made embryonic stem cell research obsolete and then called on Congress to pass a comprehensive cloning ban, ensuring as he put it, 'that all life is treated with the dignity it deserves.'" - Family Research Council, Press Release, President Tony Perkins, http://www.frc.org*

I had some thoughts of my own based on some reading I am doing on this topic. My interest is due to the relevance the subject of embryonic stem cell research has to Parkinson's Plus and other neuro-degenerative diseases. In fact, the scientists them-selves do not recommend the reaction the President had to this "discovery" and there is reason for caution. Allow me to explain.

The research related to taking skin cells and producing cells to be implanted in the brain of patients with neuro-degenerative diseases is still in the rudimentary stages and will not be effective for a minimum of 15 years. In addition, there is concern about the use of these skin cells producing a form of cancer in the brain and this problem must be solved prior to any testing which will eventually include humans.

This means that embryonic stem cells may still be critically important as a possible source of treatment for people with Alzheimer's, Diabetes, Parkinson's Disease and spinal cord injuries, in the present tense. I would pose a question: If President Bush thought stem cells were not ethical as a medical solution, *why did he sign legislation a number of years ago that allows this research to go on in a limited number of lines that were already in existence at the time of that legislation?* Pro-Life includes saving the lives of people suffering from chronic, debilitating diseases such as neuro-degenerative conditions. Those of us who have a brain disease, such as Parkinson's Plus and Parkinson's Disease, can't afford to wait fifteen years. The sufferers of these diseases are also entitled to be "treated with the dignity (they) deserve," to use a phrase the FRC coined.

In an article in *Newsweek* Magazine, in the Dec. 3, 2007 issue, entitled, "Reality Check on an Embryonic Debate," by Sharon Begley, the author seemingly explains that the President's interpretation is inaccurate. She reports that the scientists conducting the very research the President was referring to

"call the claim that reprogrammed stem cells eliminate the need for embryonic stem cells a 'serious mistake'."

Ms. Begley went on to explain that

> "it would be years before scientists understand repro-
> grammed stem cells. Applications of stem-cell science
> would be indefensibly delayed if [this research] is pursued
> at the expense of further human embryonic stem-cell re-
> search."

I think that progress being made in studying the use of skin cells as a source of stem cells with the potential to cure disease, even if rudimentary, is still vital and necessary. However, the reaction of the President and others is premature, if not unrealistic, with all of the factors being taken into account.

Diagnostic Impatience

Since I developed a movement disorder, I often find myself in contemplation. I am attempting to work out in my mind the realization of what is happening in my brain and body, and trying to process it—humanly and spiritually. Sometimes I am better able to do one or the other or both, and at other times it is not so simple. My excellent neurologist has added a medication to my regimen to aid me in dealing with the depression that arises, not just as a by-product, but as another symptomatic manifestation of my illness. Progressive Supranuclear Palsy is the most likely of the PD Plus Syndromes for me to have, and has come up with the doctor several times now over the past year. I have read much literature, particularly on-line, and many sources point out how similar Multiple Systems Atrophy and PSP are to one another. When I read of the many symptoms each can develop, it is not hard to believe how this overlapping similarity is possible, because so many are shared or are similar.

Progressive Supranuclear Palsy

No patient has all of the listed symptoms, as is true with Parkinson's. Also, it is important to remember that some symptoms arise later in the illness, or not at all, depending on the case. So no list is an ironclad criteria. For example, in PSP, the eyes will typically begin to lose their range of motion downward, and in some case, upward movements are the first to be restricted. However, eventually the eyes may become fixed in a straight forward direction, limiting vision to the immediate view which is right in front of the patient. Some sources have said that this symptom of eye movement difficulty begins to appear in the fourth year after diagnosis, on the average. In my case, I began to notice eye movement issues in the first year, which contributed to my neurologist's indication that PSP was the most likely of the Parkinson's Plus syndromes to be my diagnosis.

The Drive to "Know"

Confusing? Oh, yes! I find this information helpful to know and understand, which is due to my teacher/administrator personality, and drives me to seek to know and understand. This is how I cope—study reality, work to accept it (not resign to it) and then press on to live in the light of my faith and the love of family. The meaningfulness of life is unchanged; to the contrary, the meaningful purpose of life is *enhanced* by the realization of the preciousness of life and the fragility of human existence. Love is not love that is not in response to a choice to feel ambivalence or loathing. The same is true with the will to surge forward in living after a diagnosis of serious illness—it can be an energy-providing motivation. In my human frailty this is what I seek to do, not all the time, and never in perfect rhythm, but I attempt it nonetheless.

Dystonia

Neck pain is something that I have had a great deal of lately, due to the auto accident in which our family's mini-van was rear-ended while stuck in traffic on the freeway. Dystonia, which involves neck twisting postures, head jerking tremor, and neck pain/stiffness, are expected in my Parkinson's Plus condition.

With the accident came another challenge to add to the discomfort of these conditions—pain. I had an MRI by the treating doctor. The results of the MRI indicated that I have four disc bulges, with the range of mild to borderline severe. They progress from 1 mm to 4 mm, with the worst being at the C6-7 level (this is the lower part of the Cervical level, as it is in the area of the upper back). So these results mean that there is a logical reason why I have been experiencing even more stiffness and have had pain in my neck, upper back and shoulder.

These are challenges that can be dealt with through the physical therapy that our doctor provided for us, gentle stretching exercises and rest. Next, I will be evaluated by an orthopedist to determine if there will be any additional treatment recommended.

Neuro-Degeneration Takes a Toll

You would think that once I had gone through the initial two-and-a-half years of the process of accepting the circumstances surrounding my life that I would be resigned to it. I think it is the nature of the disease that makes the grief, loss, and acceptance cycle more difficult to grasp. A movement disorder is complex because it doesn't just take your physical abilities and gradually diminish them over time. It also involves neuro-degeneration, which means you are facing a gradual loss of brain function affecting not just abilities to move, swallow, speak and walk, but you are facing the potential of losing autonomic functions. This is true of Parkinson's Disease as well as atypical parkinsonism, particularly with regard to Parkinson's Plus syndromes. This is where the concerns linger and affect me, almost constantly.

It is hard to get these thoughts out of my consciousness because not a day goes by that I don't notice that things are changing, sometimes gradually, and other times dramatically. I have noticed that my hands are assuming awkward postures, curling into fists when I sit. When I walk, my hands raise at my sides, with my fingers spreading or curling into odd positions. I have a walking gait that is uncoordinated and forces me to march if I choose to pick up my feet, or if I don't, I am left with a shuffling, foot-dragging walking style.

Sometimes my hands have a mind of their own, with my right hand in particular suddenly raising above my elbow and flapping from my wrist, rapidly. As near as I can detect, this is what my neurologist has referred to as Chorea movements. I have written previously about what Chorea is and how it is that I would have this condition.

My neck often twists to one side or arches back. My eyes pop open wide, while my mouth goes into a frowning posture, giving the impression of grumpiness or disinterest. Still another facial expression I have looks like I have just smelled something awful. I am aware of these facial expressions when I am in public and it is hard to overcome the concern about how people will react.

Some things that are occurring are more personal and I am not ready to discuss here. Suffice to say, I have noticed some changes with regard to autonomic factors. I am also thankful that these symptoms are not worse and we are able to make adjustments that help me to forge ahead.

I am struggling to remain motivated, which is so unlike me. I am fighting ambivalence toward my music and writing. I know that the neurological effects of depression and anxiety are both taking a toll on me and interfering with these interests that typically drive me. Additionally, my hands have less control so guitar playing and typing are more of a struggle, physically. I do have a voice-activated software which is very useful in writing verbally.

I am not choosing to give in nor do I see these issues as a static situation. Maybe my sharing these thoughts openly will help someone else to feel less alone or to reflect on their problems in a new way. I have spent my life with an emphasis on Christian faith, as both my purpose and inspiration. These challenges bring doubts to the surface in a way that I haven't ever faced quite as much. I know this—God is real to me and He has shown me that He loves me.

Desiring a More Specific Diagnosis

It seems I am no closer today than I was in the past at knowing my specific diagnosis. To date, I have an "Extrapyramidal Disorder," and also an "Abnormal Involuntary Movement Disorder." That is quite a mouthful and should suffice, but my condition was also defined as one of the Parkinson's Plus syndromes, of which there are a number. I have outlined and defined these atypical Parkinson's conditions many times and there is information available in earlier pages if you need further clarification.

The reality is that each disorder takes on a definite character, in time, with enough progression of disabling symptoms. It is not uncommon for these diseases to take years to become defined in a more specific manner. I have come to accept this, although on occasion, my family and I grow impatient as we wait and wonder. The progressiveness of the condition I have is apparent to my family, friends and me. As the symptoms unfold and with continued testing and clinical observation by my neurologist, my diagnosis will narrow to a single focal point.

I have to continue to resolve to accept this uncertainty and the unknown about what my struggle will be like at a later time. The disease will define itself as it brings whatever additional challenges my way that I do not have to deal with today. That is the good news. Not knowing exactly which Parkinson's Plus syndrome I have, with Progressive Supranuclear Palsy being one of the most likely designations, means that the associated symptoms aren't well enough defined to provide that answer. So you see, I find this problem of not knowing for certain an acceptable status for the time being. I don't believe that my treatment or what things could be done medically would be altered considerably as a result of this knowledge.

During the moments when I feel compelled to know, to understand fully what I face, it seems to stem from a feeling of incompleteness or disappointment. I want to know and move on with that discovery behind me. I want my family to know so that they don't have to wonder about the nature of the illness or its cause. I have read about and heard from a number of people who have been diagnosed with a specific Parkinson's Plus disease. I know of others whose condition took years to be determined. A few have told me of their loved ones waiting many years before they were specifically diagnosed, and others whose husband, wife or parent never received a definitive answer while they were living. This is a reality I have to be prepared to face and accept.

I share this because it is an underlying truth about who I am and how I feel, thus relating to everything about the purpose of this book. The irony is that I have done my homework and am able to provide definition and clarity about the Parkinson's Plus conditions and PD itself for others, but when it comes to my case, I have to be able to satisfy my need to know with the understanding that it is not clear yet in my case. I progressed quickly and have been told what I have is "so much more than

Parkinson's Disease." I know that means it is faster progressing and involves additional disabling factors.

In the meantime, I am doing pretty well in that I am appreciating each day and doing my best to live life with passion and hope. In light of the fact that other patients with Parkinson's Plus are somewhat hard to come by, I find I am able to relate to those who have Parkinson's Disease. Sometimes this brings confusion because my condition is dissimilar to idiopathic PD in many ways. However, I do fit into the family of those who have Parkinson's Disease, as it is a movement disorder that has overlap with Parkinson's Plus. My wife and I participate in two Parkinson's Support groups for that reason. These are friends we enjoy, count on and find mutual support with as we attend meetings. Sometimes, I do realize that my case is different and wonder how it is that I am the one who has a relatively unique situation.

In life, sometimes questions remain and answers do not come. We have to be able to accept those times, if we have done our best and have run out of immediate solutions. Finding peace with that isn't easy to accomplish, but it is the best conclusion to a persistent, unanswerable dilemma.

Parkinson's Plus Continues to Confuse

Staying Active

In the third year of my condition, I had a wonderful opportunity to visit another regional Parkinson's Support Group as a guest presenter. In spite of the symptoms I have from Parkinson's Plus, including difficulties that interfere with my speech, eye movements and a constantly moving and twisting body, I still enjoy being able to share with friends about what has happened, what is occurring now, and where this condition is taking me. My music is, at times, compromised by a lack of fine motor coordination and strength, as well as vocal changes that affect my voice. Still, I did share some songs, along with telling my story. Those present showed appreciation and Karrie and I enjoyed visiting this group immensely! This is an example of what I referred to in my song entitled, "I Will Go On." There is much to live for and I can still serve. If you doubted that you could, as a Parkinsonism patient or otherwise, you need to think about how your background, talents, hobbies, or former career provide avenues for you to continue on in your life.

Parkinson's Plus a Misunderstood Term

Parkinson's Plus, like all movement disorders, impacts a person across the board. It is difficult to clarify the distinguishing features of PD Plus, in light of the name that has been given these various syndromes, including Multiple Systems Atrophy, Progressive Supranuclear Palsy, Lewy Body Disease, and Corticobasal Ganglionic Degeneration, to name several more prevalent versions. In my case, I have a number of observable aspects that are comparable to idiopathic PD. These are specifically: tremors, dyskinesia, facial masking and slow, imbalanced movements. Lately the dyskinesia is more pronounced. This takes the form of random, twisting, turning movements of my trunk, legs, neck, wrists, and fingers. I get into awkward postures and tilt my head to one side while my face is blank or frowning in appearance. This is also part of Dystonia, teaming up with dyskinesia to create some bothersome and awkward public moments.

Parkinson's Plus Contrasted with PD

The biggest question I get from Parkinson's Disease patients is, "How is Parkinson's Plus really different from Parkinson's Disease?" A very good question and I will give a brief written reply here. Keep in mind, my goal in this book is to write things that are relevant, understandable for all of us, and focused more on clarity than medical terminology. I will leave that to the professionals: neurologists, movement disorder specialists and research scientists in the great Universities. Parkinson's Disease has four hallmark categories of symptoms: Slowness of Movement (bradykinesia), Resting Tremor (is worst when the individual is still, at rest), Postural Instability (balance problems caused by brain dysfunction), and Rigidity of Joints/Muscles. There are many other symptoms and medical issues that result from Parkinson's Disease and they range from swallowing difficulty to speech troubles and even a masked facial expression, to name some but nowhere near all of the troubling problems. Forty percent of Parkinson's patients will struggle with dementia to one extent or another. If you were to look for visual cues in the case of a Parkinson's Plus patient, you might see a number of these outward signs manifested, so what is the difference?

How My Case Progressed

Parkinson's Plus has been called "Parkinson's on Steroids" by a close friend I have known since high school. That is a humorous, but all too poignant description. The word "Parkinson's" in the disease name is misleading, in a number of ways, and causes confusion to those around the Parkinson's Plus patient. Parkinson's Plus does include a number of the symptoms listed above, but in most cases these increase in severity at an alarmingly faster pace, and will become disabling much sooner. Parkinson's Plus has such a variety of forms, so I will give you examples from my own experience. Balance became a problem for me within a few months of my first visit to the doctor to find out why I had tremors that were increasing in amplitude. I noticed that I would sway whenever I tried to stand in one place. I had the sense that I might begin to fall, and often I would fight to steady myself. Walking became a difficult chore, with an uncoordinated gait, causing my legs to be hard to control and my arms awkwardly curled up and hanging at my sides, and a reduced "arm swing" to give me balance. All of this occurs involuntarily and gives one the feeling that their body is someone else's. My eyes pop wide open at times, and at others they close involuntarily. My eye movements are somewhat limited, so that I have to turn my head directly toward a speaker in order to focus on them without pain. The muscles governing my mouth and voice are slow and stiffened so that speech is interrupted, slow and muffled. I have tremors, but what makes it unique from Parkinson's Disease is that they involve my entire body, with a constant rhythmic tremor in my trunk, affecting my head, neck, arms, and legs on both sides of my body.

Specific Similarities and Differences

Parkinson's Disease classically affects a single side of the body, initially, and eventually affects both sides after a number of years. Parkinson's Plus begins by causing tremors, stiffness and a lack of coordination on both sides, symmetrically. Parkinson's Disease has a more gradual onset of symptoms while Parkinson's Plus dramatically increases in severity, noticeably fast. From the onset of tremors in the summer of 2005, I was disabled from my career by the following February of 2006. Although I don't want to over generalize, or say that some cases of Parkinson's Disease don't have an accelerated onset, this is not typically the case. Levodopa in the form of "Sinemet" is often used to treat tremors, rigidity and other large motor movement issues in Parkinson's Disease. Levodopa is highly effective in Parkinson's Disease, giving the doctor an important marker to determine the diagnosis of Parkinson's Disease. In my case, it was apparent that, although taking Levodopa, I would not get rid of my tremors completely, ever. In idiopathic PD, the tremors will cease for several hours; in my case they are lessened, but never gone. At times, my body will be moving and tremors prevalent as though I have taken no Levodopa, though I have not missed a dose. Sinemet (Levodopa) is beneficial to me, helping me to move less slowly, and decreasing the tremor enough to steady my hand a bit so I can type or play guitar. It also helps my outlook to be more balanced and this is really helpful for those around me.

Parkinson's Plus causes a quicker onset and a more severe problem of balance, making walking and standing more difficult. In regular PD, most patients remain ambulatory for a number of years, with walking eventually becoming more and more difficult. Freezing will cause a Parkinson's Disease patient to temporarily get stuck in one place, or even fall down, causing injury. Parkinson's Plus will affect the Cerebellum and the brain stem, depending on the specific disease, causing standing with balance to be difficult and making the walking pattern nearly impossible. I require a wheelchair to shop in a store or visit a baseball game, because walking is not manageable in a bigger venue such as these. I can still use the cane to get out of the car and go into Starbucks, one of the favorite activities my wife and I like to do together.

Many with Parkinson's Disease will remain employed or at work for a number of years, and keep driving for a good long time, as well. I was forced to end my career within five months of onset, and my driving freedom ended, simultaneously. My cognition slowed, my speech became interrupted and halting, and I had trouble with depression and standing, all in the first few months. These things did not allow me the luxury of a self-determined exit from a thirty-year career in public schools. I cannot tell you how much I have missed the days at school, the students, the teachers, parents in the community, the support and maintenance staff, and the fellow administrators and managers. It was difficult to give that all up. Parkinson's Plus moved in quickly, aggressively and changed so many aspects of my life almost overnight.

Parkinson's Plus has an average prognosis of death after 7–10 years, where Parkinson's Disease typically has a slower progression and does not always mean a shorter life span for the affected patient. Parkinson's Plus diseases interfere with breathing and swallowing in a much quicker progression. Those with Shy Drager have autonomic failures and face very serious medical issues. Falling may become an overwhelming threat, particularly for those who have Progressive Supranuclear Palsy. As the Parkinson's Plus patient progresses at a faster rate, they are immobilized, causing increasingly serious health problems, as a result.

I have an ever progressing lack of coordination, cognitive difficulties are becoming more evident with memory and decision-making effects, and my eyes are becoming more difficult to move. The key to all of this is that the Parkinson's Plus conditions do, in fact, affect the movement center of the brain. This area, called the Basal Ganglia, is the key region of impairment in the brain of the Parkinson's Disease patient. The Parkinson's Plus patient has this and *other areas of the brain also degenerating*, and these areas are those that affect other movement and bodily functions, as well as cognition. Thus the *Plus* in Parkinson's Plus.

In Conclusion

"Parkinson's Disease on steroids," indeed. Each patient with a movement disorder is facing great difficulty. As another friend quipped, "It is not a picnic," either way. Parkinson's Plus means the struggles will generally come faster and will limit the individual in their life goals and abilities much more aggressively. To really break this topic down, go back to chapter three where I have described specific diseases in layman's terms, but in much more detail. *The word "Parkinson's" in "Parkinson's Plus," is somewhat misleading. These diseases are distinct from each other, as my wife explains.* When I am further diagnosed at some point, I will be able to hang a more specific label on my condition. In the meantime, my treatment is on target and wouldn't be noticeably different. My neurologist addresses all of my needs and does it well. So, I don't require a more specific subgroup name.

Going On in Life

Suffice it to say, I am going to keep on making the best of every day and give what I am able. Music and writing are those things that I can do in addition to the most important, spending time with my family. We have a great family and frequently get together to talk, eat and laugh. Church gives me the spiritual balance—and there is much support and love in that environment—which is an abundant blessing. Looking at these factors, I conclude with this statement, "I am a lucky guy!"

Chapter Five:

PD Plus Me Blog - Reader's Responses and Stories

I N THIS CHAPTER I have included my written correspondences with individuals I met electronically through the "PD Plus Me" blog. The stories within this chapter are from real people who have been touched by reading the blog or have had specific experiences of their own that they are generously sharing here for the benefit of the reader. I found these messages, stories, remembrances and poems to be uplifting and inspiring. I am sure that you will, as well. I have used first names only, out of respect for the writer's privacy. In some cases, a second party mentioned in an email has been given a pseudonym. My sincere thanks to each contributor.

Looking for those with Parkinson's Plus and PD

I have so many thoughts today, having stepped back for a week without writing on this blog. I am increasingly aware of the uniqueness of Parkinson's Plus, in that there is not enough information about the cause and there are less resources available than are more easily found on the topic of idiopathic Parkinson's

Disease. I find that in that rare instance where I am able to be in contact with someone else who is facing a diagnosis of Parkinson's Plus, whichever the particular subtype, that it is a gift that is indescribable. I find that others are facing similar issues of postural instability, speech difficulty, over-reactive startle response, walking issues, eye dysfunctions, cognitive slowing, and mood difficulties. In addition, Parkinson's Plus patients are troubled by medications, that although are effective in treating PD, they do not last long enough or are inconsistent in their medical benefit for the "plus" patient.

These patients are out there and are in need of others who understand and might help them to make sense of all of these changes. *I am here as a resource for any such person and I want to extend my willingness to communicate, offer support, give ideas on contacts and support groups, or just to be a friend who understands.* I am very blessed when such an opportunity arises through my blog, in a support group I attend or in an on-line Yahoo message board group where a forum of ideas such as these are more plentiful.

I know that stopping a progressive disease is a tall order, if not highly unlikely, but we can make the best of our days and be available to assist others facing a similar plight. That thought gives me an energy little else does.

If you are surfing by and find this site, and are sharing a commonality with me in the fight against neuro-degenerative diseases, particularly movement disorders, please drop me a line, make a comment on this blog or send me your *diagnosis biography* so that I might share it with others. You may make a difference in someone's life that you had not thought possible. I would love to hear your story and publish it on-line.

Your friend in the struggle– Dan

Reader's Story - My Mother's Fight with PSP

The following is a true to life account of Donna, one of my blog readers, describing the experiences she had while supporting her beloved mother, Darlene, as she faced Progressive Supranuclear Palsy with courage and perseverance.

My mom (Darlene) started having symptoms of something amiss as far back as 1996. Her toes would wiggle on their own, which progressed into a leg tremor over that year and the next. This usually happened when she was at rest, but not asleep. This produced an early diagnosis of Restless Leg Syndrome.

By early 1997, she started shuffling when she walked and had some moments of lost balance. As that year progressed she would fall a number of times, none seriously. Her golf game suffered though! Doctors began then suggesting she visit a type of doctor that is similar to a physical therapist but not exactly (I simply cannot remember this doctor)! There were many non-invasive tests and muscle strengthening protocols.

In 1998, she experienced a number of mood changes and some personality changes, too. She was quick to bicker and seemed unable to concentrate. She was usually a very outgoing person, extremely quick-witted, but she became argumentative in a way she never had been before. Her doctor sent her to a psychiatrist who said she was "depressed." Around this time, a neurologist at Ohio State University was consulted for the first time who claimed that she was in need of a "Posterior Cervical Laminectomy". The theory (as I remember it) was that by removing calcium deposits on the back of her spine in the neck area, her balance would return and the leg tremor would cease. As you might guess, we proceeded with the surgery and neither improvement was realized: quite the contrary, since the surgery proved very difficult for her and recovery was very hard. I kick myself still for allowing this surgery with so little research, but I know hindsight is 20/20.

In 1999, she discovered breast cancer, which was totally un-related to her neurological conditions but nonetheless a set-back. She underwent another surgery for a simple mastectomy; no chemo or radiation and returned to life "cancer free." By this time, she was having some vision problems that, coupled with the balance issues, caused her to stop driving. This loss of inde-pendence was a major blow for a 59 year-old woman. Another neurologist from OSU was consulted in late 1999 and he men-tioned PSP for the first time, but it was not a diagnosis per se.

At that time, she and her husband relocated to Tennessee where they built a retirement home and planned to golf their lives away, quite happily. Of course, by the time they moved in the fall of 1999, Mom's balance made golfing prohibitive. By 2000, she was falling frequently even with the use of a rolling walker. She suffered a broken arm, a broken nose, and stitches in her head on more than one occasion. What we perceived as stubbornness (a family trait she held in spades!) seemed to pre-vent her from learning that she could no longer get up and go as she wanted. Again, hindsight tells me that it was simply PSP preventing her from learning.

That summer, July 2000, she went to the emergency room from choking on some food—the beginning of serious difficul-ties swallowing. She was unable to really control her bladder, although this, too, had been somewhat of a problem prior. She refused to wear Depends or anything at this point. Her neurolo-gist at Vanderbilt was unsure of a diagnosis and never settled on anything. We switched to a doctor at the University of Ten-nessee and the neurologist there ruled out PSP on the basis of her "lack of axial rigidity." True, Mom had a good bit of mobil-ity in her arms, legs and neck in 2000-2001, but she had every other sign of PSP, including the inability to move the eyes down-ward. By this time, after more research, I was already convinced. She was prescribed Sinemet, Amantadine and other drugs I've forgotten along the way. I attended the symposium on PSP in Baltimore, hosted by the CurePSP organization, and again felt confident that it was indeed the disease.

All these symptoms progressed over 2001 and 2002. By the summer of 2002, she was moved to a wheelchair. She had some numbness and weakness in the left hand that made moving the wheelchair difficult. Her eyesight was fair, but directing the eyes was increasingly hard to do. She had bursts of laughter and crying at strange times and almost overnight her voice turned to a whisper. At this time, her husband felt unable to care for her at home in Tennessee and they agreed a nursing home was the best move. I insisted this be one near me in Atlanta and she moved here in July 2002. This was a VERY difficult transition but I still believe a necessary one.

Neurologists at Emory considered PSP, as well as Multiple System Atrophy (MSA) and Olivopontocerebellar Atrophy (OPCA). Eventually, they settled on PSP. Of course, every six months we would visit again and be told with greater certainty each time that we were most likely dealing with PSP, and there was nothing really to be done. Eventually, Mom was taking Artane for the tremor which was a great benefit. She started Namenda as well, but that didn't provide much benefit. She was also on anti-depressants (Zoloft) and was taking Aricept, as well. That combination became the accepted protocol that she remained on (with few variations) from 2002 until her death in 2006.

From 2002 through 2004 she gradually lost the ability to move her eyes where she wanted and to look downward at all. Her face became a mask, almost a grimace, most of the time. She became unable to speak very well by mid-2003 but had bursts of sentences. However, if one paid close attention and listened closely, she was definitely able to communicate through 2004. Most people, of course, didn't spend the proper time and it was very frustrating for her to interact with people who clearly thought she was uninterested or unable to understand them, while neither was true. Although we saw some cognitive slowing at this time, for the most part, her mind remained sharp throughout her life.

2005 brought many difficulties as she lost the ability to swallow and to speak. We came up with a means of communication whereby she would raise one finger to indicate "yes" and two fingers to indicate "no." I became an expert at conducting complete two-sided conversations based entirely on yes or no answers. When she tired of this she would sometimes choose a particular middle finger to get me to shut up and we would both laugh. Her sense of humor remained intact! She refused pureed foods throughout her life as well as a feeding tube, decisions which I supported. While I didn't necessarily agree with the pureed food issue, I did support her decision and made sure it was carried out. I never felt like my mom was unable to make decisions for herself, ever. She simply needed a voice and this was a role I gladly filled.

Later in the same year, she had developed a great deal of rigidity and would often find herself stuck in odd postures. Some days her back would be arched and she would be looking at the sky, unable to move her head. Other days, she would be tilted to one side but with a stiff neck that prohibited her head from moving much. She never shied away from a trip, though, and I continued taking her on walks and bringing her to my house to spend Saturday and Sunday. With help she could stand and walk a few tentative steps from chair to car, etc.

We always felt the disease brought many plateaus. She would find herself with a certain level of ability, then experience a decline of some sort, often triggered by an illness or a fall or some incident that happened. This would bring a new plateau and no changes for a while. Oddly enough, in January 2006, for whatever reason, she experienced a short improvement. Almost overnight, she found herself more fluid in her movements in her neck and, most importantly, able to speak almost in full sentences and fairly loudly. This lasted about 10 days and it was such a joy! We were able to discuss many things and talk almost normally. Those few things that we were never able to clarify in the past year (when 1 finger or 2 wouldn't work) were suddenly clarified and we were both relieved. It was so strange! As quickly as it came, however, one day it was gone and we were back where we were.

In February 2006, she had her first bout of aspiration pneumonia and it took its toll. She was down to about 110 pounds now, although she had been 170 pounds when she moved into the nursing home. Her strength was minimal. In early March, we believe she suffered a stroke or mini-strokes, and she suddenly lost use of her left arm, entirely. It also greatly affected her swallowing and she began having great difficulty eating at all. On March 10, 2006 she was rushed to the ER again with thoughts of a stroke as she suddenly lost use of her left leg entirely. The next day she could stand on the leg again, with help, but by the 18th, again, the leg wouldn't work at all. By this date, she was barely able to swallow and the nurses did a great job of offering food and water, yet standing by to suction her throat if needed. She again developed aspiration pneumonia and we knew then she couldn't fight it. On March 20 her pupils were at odds – one very large and dilated, the other a pinpoint; but, she was able to communicate with me somewhat and I knew that she was "there." However, on the 21st, she slept all day and did not get out of bed. On the 23rd, she was up out of her bed and in the wheelchair, still with oxygen, but she knew we were there with her. On the 24th, again, she seemed almost out of consciousness and remained that way until she passed away quietly the evening of March 26th. We were all there– her sister, me, my one and two-year-old daughters, and my husband—and we continued to talk to her to ease her transition. I always prayed she would leave this life peacefully and it gives me great comfort to know she did so, in my arms, and that now she is at peace. – Donna

Reader's Story of Mother's Experience with PSP - Revisited

Below is a follow up from the writer of the article immediately above, entitled, "Reader's Story - My Mother's Fight with PSP." Here she comments regarding the frustration of her mother, Darlene, as she hoped for a definitive diagnosis.

I have recently stopped in to your blog again and felt the need to reach out to you. Your post yesterday where you recognize the power of not naming your condition really spoke to me. You'll remember my mom had PSP, and she was continually frustrated by the inability to define the disease. With each doctor appointment you could see the hope in her eyes that perhaps THIS TIME they would definitively say "You have _____" (fill in with a disease name). Even if the answer was indeed PSP, she felt that somehow just knowing its name would give her comfort. Of course, with most appointments she was disappointed that this magical diagnosis didn't occur. I wish I could've read your words back then, because I think it really would have helped her! Since the treatments are virtually the same, the best course of action is to focus on those, get excellent care, and enjoy life and relationships. You are right on track!

Congratulations, too, on getting through your MRI – I know that is a tough one. I wanted to also share this link that I received some months back that you might find interesting.

http://radpod.org/2007/02/23/progressive-supranuclear-palsy/

It shows an MRI of the brain of a person with PSP. When you click on the image itself, it will superimpose a penguin on a certain area of the brain. This is the first time I had heard of this "penguin sign" and have never seen anything else written about it. Perhaps your neurologist would find it interesting.

Again, my best to you and your family, as always.

Your friend, Donna

Reply to Donna

Hi Donna,

It was so encouraging to hear from you and to read your thoughts of support and confirmation of the things I am trying to grasp about PSP as we go along in the process. Your insights from a perspective of living through this with your mother are so valuable to me and as you can imagine, quite a rare opportunity for me and my family.

I understand what your mother was feeling back then. I have the same desire: to just know the name to hang on this and then I can go off into the sunset. But, alas, it isn't a realistic expectation and as you and I have discussed, it won't necessarily change the prognosis and/or drug treatment.

The imaging with the penguin was very interesting. I am going to do some of my own research about this concept and patterning of midbrain effect.

It is so awesome to have someone who knows where we are going and cares. Stay in touch Donna – Dan

A Follow-up Comment from Donna

Dan,

As usual, I find your site and your thoughts quite moving! I would add to your comments as a note to all caregivers, please allow your loved ones (the patients) to express themselves too, even if that means giving a good shoulder to cry on. My one regret in how I handled my Mom's PSP was that I so badly wanted her to have a good day and to be happy that I think I "entertained" too much. I planned outings, read to her, talked incessantly about the news of the day...anything to get a laugh or a smile. I don't regret that part, but I rarely let her just have time to cry with me, even though I cried often by myself about what was happening to her. I am so grateful for your perspective and your words of thanks to your wife and all caregivers. It is very comforting to me, even now, two years after my Mom has passed. You have a gift for communication that is a blessing to us all!

Best regards,
Donna

Response to Donna

Donna,

Thank you for your feedback and much support. Your story, posted here previously, has been a great blessing and provided insight to many. I am sure that you providing both meaningful experiences, and a shoulder to cry on, were both appreciated mightily by your mother. Bless you for the person you are and for letting others get a glimpse of the experiences you have gone through. – Dan

Comment from Mark H.

Dan,

I have asked myself on several occasions if I would be able to handle Dan's situation as well as he continues to do so. In all honesty, I fear not. It causes me to question my faith, my inner strength, and even my manhood. A test of your magnitude would, I believe, expose a cowardice that embarrasses me to ponder....Mark H.

Reply to Mark H.
Mark H,

I think that your courage comes through your honesty. It is so hard to find transparency like yours in the world. As far as facing the situation, you will never know what friends like you mean. You have personally given me your strength many times. I thank you.

Dan

More Inspiration from Mark H.
Dan,

For many of us, your daily struggles have reminded those of us more fortunate at the moment, to be grateful for all that we are blessed with in our own lives. Every time I get a little down or frustrated, I think of Karrie and you. Those thoughts get me back to reality and help me move forward quickly. I owe you more than you can imagine. We'll be seeing you soon...Mark H.

Replying to Mark
Mark,

Sometimes you put thoughts into words in a way that no one else can. You are an example of those that have supported this site since it began 17 months ago, as well as supporting our family through it all. I am still appreciating and enjoying the Dragon Naturally Speaking software you provided. I do look forward to seeing you both!

Dan

More Mark H.
Dan,

You've never been so concise and pointedly right on the money. Thank you for being a friend who has helped to bring peace, contentment, and joy to my soul. I am grateful for the years that I have known Karrie and you. My life couldn't possibly have been the same without the two of you....Mark H. *(This note was a reference to the article, "Can God Redeem Any Circumstance?" This is found in Chapter Six, "With Faith I Will Go On.")*

Response to Mark H.

Mark H, Your friendship means every bit as much to us! We have treasured knowing you these many years. Your feedback on this blog has been so consistently there, and your emotional and practical support during the PD Plus years has been a Godsend. Thank you for sharing your writing with us these last two years.

Dan

From Bernice
Hello Dan,

I am glad we are friends, also. You have helped me gain some peace with this disease as much as I have helped you.

And I, like you, wonder when we see so much predictability in the progression, why we can't intercept it somewhere along the way.

I am so happy it is helping in your desire to walk more closely with God. It certainly had that effect on Ken and me.

I wanted to share with you the comments of Ru, whose husband is also stricken with this disease. I shared with her your blog address and asked her to read what you had posted recently about your church attendance. Here are comments she sent me today.

From Ru, as referred to by Bernice

Dear Bernice,

This is amazing and it did most certainly bring tears to my eyes...I listened to the music, too, and read Dan's background. What a remarkable man and what a shame, but I try to believe that God has better use for people in the condition they find themselves...shuttering as I say that! For we know not what is ahead for us! Are you subscribed to his blogspot? I don't know much about blogs and all these new things that are popping up everywhere. I'd love to download some of his music. It is beautiful. Is it necessary to subscribe? – Ru

More from Bernice

Dan, This lady is a faithful caregiver to Will her husband. They live in Alabama. Will is further advanced in the disease than you but she has managed to keep him at home. She does have some help come in at least once a week for a few hours so she can get out. But she has also been caring for a mother, whom she has just placed in an assisted living place. She has had her plate full, but is a good Christian woman and carrying it with grace and dignity. And she has a terrific sense of humor in spite of it all that she maintains most of the time. We hope to meet in person one day soon. But we write each other almost daily.

Thank you for keeping in touch. And I pray you and Karrie have a blessed day.

Your sister in Christ, Bernice

Dear Dan,

I hope you don't mind me passing on some of the things you write to my friends. I was so impressed with what you wrote about your experience in church I told several of my friends to read it and I am passing along to you some of their comments. You can see by that the impression you are making on different people. This man who wrote the following is a man who provides medical equipment - i.e., wheelchairs, walkers, van lifts, etc. For disabled people free of charge. He started a foundation called "Friends of Disabled Adults and Children" in 1986 in Atlanta (www.Fodac.org) fixing a few wheelchairs in his garage and giving them away.

They have now given away over 19,000 wheelchairs, along with much other medical equipment. His wife has passed away and he has since retired and moved to SC. He is a very good friend of mine, and is still actively involved in this kind of ministry. Just this morning he wrote me the following:

"I am going up to NC to do an assessment for a scooter and a van lift for a woman with a neuromuscular disease. It is a bit far but not too bad. The husband cried when I told him I would give it all to him."

Anyway, his comments about your work are below.

From Ed, as referred to by Bernice

Dear Bernice:

   This is an incredible piece of work. Part of the tragedy of diseases and injuries is that we will never know what that person could have become had they been spared this fate. There is a school of thought that such folks are moved by their experience to reach these heights but a more reasonable approach is that their potential is limited by their disease. Dan is an anomaly, a man who knows what is happening to his body but is not mentally destroyed by those effects.

   God bless him as he has blessed us all.

   Love, Ed

From Ru to Bernice

Bernice,

   I just had to tell you about what happened earlier this afternoon. Some people might not think much about it, but because you sent Dan's blog, I was able to use some of his comments to comfort my next door neighbor or her sister.

   Mrs. O is probably 76 or so and she lost her husband about two years ago. She keeps an immaculate house and her yards are manicured. She loves flowers and stayed in the yard more than inside when weather permitted. But, she was always unhappy with life, or so it seemed. She's been a good neighbor as far as not "bothering" anyone but lives in her own world which seems to be focused on keeping up her yards. We've been "yard friends" for the eight years we've lived here and that's about it. Her husband, Mr. F, was a real gentleman and seemed so sweet.

A few weeks ago Mrs. O fell and fractured her foot or vice versa. She had to wear a boot and, a couple of weeks later, I saw her out pulling weeds without a boot, so I figured, "Well, must not be as bad as she thought." Anyhow, I learned two weeks ago that she'd gone for a mammogram and they found a lump, which she has since had removed. But the doctor says the cancer is in her bones, which made me wonder why he removed the lump. On top of that it was done locally by a small-town doctor, not a specialist. Well, he is a surgeon.

I had gone over once and couldn't get anyone to the door, but today I went and her sister was there. Mrs. O and I talked a little and she wondered if she had done the right thing by not letting him remove the breast. I told her not to worry about that. She'd done what she believed to be the best at the time and she'd do the same thing when she had to make the next decision. Leave it in God's hands.

Her sister followed me to the door and I ask her exactly how things stand. She said that it was in her bones, etc., as I mentioned above. She indicated that her sister got angry, sad, prayed, cussed, but she knew she wasn't suppose to question God. When she said that, I remembered Dan's words from the Scriptures and reminded her of them. They go to church, so it wasn't like she'd never heard them ...but then, it was like she'd never heard them, if you can understand that. I told her that it was perfectly normal to have these feelings and to remember that Jesus asked God why He had forsaken Him, and that it was no sin to ask God, "Why?" The answer will come in God's time. I also told her that I go through the same questions. Why has God taken or allowed more than 8 years of my life and Will's to be sapped away with disease while there are men and women in their 80's and 90's walking around, and some are even driving? But I already know the answer: our suffering is supposed to bring honor to God. It's a testing to bring out the purity of our faith and letting God show us what He can do. I fail the test far too often. Time to get back to the test, or better yet to the studying of His Word.

Thank you for sharing the blog with me, and tell Dan to hang in there. There is purpose in his suffering! Not just for my neighbor, but for me. Maybe there is hope for me? I'm so impatient!

Love,
Ru

More From Bernice

You are welcome Dan. I have been meaning to write to you as well, and tell you I would be happy to have Ken included in your book if you are going to do a chapter on others. I also wanted to tell you that you are on our permanent prayer list in the Stephen Ministry. We all love you and are wishing and praying for the best for you and Karrie.

They all know you through me.

I must go get ingredients for a casserole for our Stephen Ministry Picnic tonight. Nice to hear from you. We are still dodging rain drops here in Michigan.

LV, Bernice

Dear Dan:

I sent your blog to another friend (Ed the one who does the wheelchairs) and he sent me some comments about it along with his last letter. I won't send it all because part of it contains confidential information but wanted you to hear his comments about your blog.

Bernice

From Ed to Bernice

Dear Bernice:

Not all pain and uncertainties are physically based. I find myself confused, hurting and deeply troubled that my actions have hurt others so deeply. They have left me emotionally scarred too, and Dan's words, which I have re-read often, help me in some mysterious way to understand my own frailties. You can't give away thousands of wheelchairs without feeling empathy for those who suffer and yet I seem to be troubled by some of my acts!

That paradox is a mystery to me too and I am struggling to understand. Dan's words help.

Thank you for sending them.

Love, Ed

A Brief Story about Bernice's Husband, Who Fought PSP Bravely
Kenneth

Submitted by Kenneth's Spouse Bernice

Kenneth was a wonderful husband, father, grandfather and a firefighter. He had his first symptoms of neurological disease in January of 1987. The first symptoms that were noticed were loss of balance, stuttering step, slight tremor off and on, micrographia and the loss of smell.

Kenneth was misdiagnosed and treated for Parkinson's from 1988 to 1994, when the neurology clinic declared he did not have Parkinson's, but they didn't know what he had. Another medical facility subsequently said it was PSP or MSA. A third health care organization finally diagnosed it definitely as PSP in

September 1995. However upon death, the brain tissue showed it was MSA rather than PSP. Since we were on the PSP list serving so long, and I learned all my information from them, I stayed with them.

He was on a feeding tube from Oct 1995 until his death in June 2000. Kenneth maintained a sense of humor, and seemed to be fully cognitive, but could not speak, or even communicate with facial expressions by then. He was quadriplegic, existing only in a wheel chair or bed. I cared for him at home with the help of a Hoyer lift, hospital bed, feeding pump, and wheel chair. He was catheterized. Also, I had a roll-in shower so I could bathe him regularly. I did not have outside help because at that time hospice told me he could only have six months, and if it ran out then they couldn't help me. I know it has changed since then, but I never knew when it would be his last 6 months so I didn't call them back. I finally did call just two weeks before he died. They came and did an intake, and then the nurse went on two week vacation. He died while she was gone.

A Poem about Kenneth, By Bernice
The Golden Cord

They look at me with heavy eyes, down-turned mouth and frown,
"My dear you must get out – away – this job will get you down."
With sighs they shake their head, rub hands across their face,
"Why don't you hire someone to come in and take your place?"
I try to smile and say I will, if I feel it's too much strain,
But just for now, I'm doing fine, there's lots more sun than rain.
They tell me what a saint I am, I'm earning my reward
I guess it is hard for them to see, the gleaming "Golden Cord."
The one that yokes your heart to mine and lightens every load

The one that never snaps or tears, or breaks along the road.
We've walked this path together for more than 40 years
Our tie grows ever stronger with the laughter and the tears.
They look upon your shuttered eyes, your hands clenched in a fist
They cannot see the treasure there, yet I feel very blessed.
What greater gift could I receive, than knowing in my mind,
God trusted me to care for you until the end of time.
How could they know the memories we hold from years gone by
The joys, the love and laughter, and the tears we both would cry.
The houses, jobs, and animals, the children —one-two-three!
The camping, fishing, hiking and the cruises on the sea.
They cannot know the pleasures of our travels far from home.
The kissing of the Blarney Stone, the Seven Hills of Rome,
The Eiffel Tower, London Bridge, The Andes in Peru
Antipode Australia, and green New Zealand, too.
And I alone can share with you those very private things
Which others deem undignified, distasteful or unclean.
I'm grateful for this mission as each new day unfolds
To know that you're well cared for, is my Olympic Gold.
They do not know, they cannot see, the gifts that we have treasured
They do not come in bank accounts or things that can be measured.
If they could see within our hearts the love that overflows
They'd know we need no pity, just a love song, and a rose.
And when that golden cord is clipped, and we walk no more together
I'll pluck some rays of memories from my former sunny weather.

And wear them in my heart, and know with God you will abide
Until we meet and once again, the golden cord is tied.

© 1997 Bernice Bowers
Used by Permission

Kenneth as a Grandfather

The following essay, written in the form of a letter, is addressed to Kenneth, the grandfather of Hailey. She was assigned to do a paper and decided that she would write about her inspiring grandfather Kenneth. Not only did she submit it for her required assignment, but she sent it as a gift to her grandfather on Father's Day. Hailey is the Granddaughter of Bernice, a friend who has supported me and so many others who participate in an online community for Parkinson's Plus and PSP patients. Hailey was 15 years old when this was written, and is now a grown woman who is a professional flight attendant. I thought others would benefit from reading about the love, respect and lessons learned through the struggles and courage of Hailey's grandfather.

Grandpa Kenneth

In the spring of 1981, my family, including my dad and mom, my twin brother, and my grandparents, took a vacation up to our lovely log cabin in Vail. That week I saw my grandpa's inner beauty. During our stay, I was 4 years old and I loved to climb to our loft on the ladder. On one occasion, I suddenly lost my grip and hit my head on the ladder cracking my skull. I can remember vividly, my grandpa caring for me. His strength and his reassuring words helped me through my accident. After this time of comfort I always believed in him.

"Let's go catch some fish, grandpa!" my twin brother and I pleaded while pulling on his arm. My brother and I always loved when our grandpa visited us. It meant he would teach us his secrets of fishing. He was the best fisherman in the world.

"Be quiet kids, or you'll scare the fish", my grandpa warned us firmly. We untied the rope and started to push off the dock. My brother and I realized we were venturing off into our own little world. A world of peace known only to us. As we steadily took off into the middle of Grand Lake, our eyes brightened with anticipation. The excitement increased when we put our bait on the hook, casting with our fishing pole and finally reeling our lines in. Most of all, I liked the attention we got, from Grandpa helping us.

At that moment, I respected my grandpa with all my heart. I knew that when we came back without fish he would not care and would still believe in us, no matter what. He was so smart, and I knew he loved us, tremendously.

Years have passed and he has long since retired. He told me of his heroic deeds of saving lives during rescues and putting out fires. My grandpa was a humble fireman for all of his life. I am so proud of my grandpa. He is a person who does not need gratitude, and who is not famous, or on the television, yet he has such a fulfilling life. He has made a difference and had an obvious purpose in life.

Although we live far away from each other, our love and strong bonding is recaptured on our short, yet meaningful visits. Such little things as teaching me how to cook a Mexican Pizza, or our joking about him pulling a wheelie in his wheelchair, mean so much to me. He has shown me a wonderful outlook on life. My grandpa has taught me that I do not have to be famous to be a worthwhile individual who makes a difference in the world.

Now my grandfather has Progressive Supranuclear Palsy. It is a rare, progressive neurological disease, which has rendered him nearly helpless. He has strength and perseverance as this disease progresses. Throughout the years it has been persistently debilitating to my grandpa. It has made this man take many steps backward in the process of trying to move forward. My admiration for him is growing stronger than ever, and I am comforted in our recent visits because it draws us closer. His phone calls hurt me to no end. This hurting starts when I hear my grandpa, who rarely showed strong emotion, break down and cry. I have learned to comfort those who need comforting from my grandpa, who has always been my comfort.

I love you Grandpa.

Your loving granddaughter,

Hailey

The above Submissions about the life of Kenneth were submitted by Bernice and are used by permission.

From Pastor Brad

Good morning, Dan. Lori and I returned Sunday night from a weekend in San Diego. Our anniversary consisted of dinner out at a good Steakhouse. Very good food, but uneventful otherwise.

When we returned we both read the updates on your blog. Your journal entry was one of the most meaningful reflections of a person's inner journey that I have ever seen. It had so many different insightful reflections. As I read it, I thought back to one of the foundational experiences of my ministry that happened about 27 years ago. There was a woman in our church named Mrs. V. Mrs. V., like you, was an extraordinary person. Part of what made her extraordinary in my mind was that she was able to describe the inner most parts of her physical and spiritual journey during her fight with cancer. I have always felt blessed beyond words because she was willing to reveal this part of life to me over the years. You, too, are doing the same for so many people.

The fact that the blog is growing says volumes about its relevance and benefits to people. It is much more than just reading the events/experiences of some external figure in life. It is a gift to people who, like you, are trying to integrate their experience with many different parts of life (physical, emotional, spiritual, family, and medical). I know that your blog is intended for people going through similar things, but I see it in much broader terms. While you're experiences are very specific, the underlying struggles are part of the human experience. Many of the questions, frustrations and growing points are common and your writing bridges across these divides. Besides all this, your writing is absolutely outstanding. You have quite a gift!

I just want you to know that many times people have far greater impact upon the lives of others than they can imagine. You are one of these people. Maybe someday you will realize this—I know others do.

With love and admiration. Brad

From Dan to Noreen

Noreen, I was so moved by the message below, that I called Karrie in and read most of it to her aloud. You touched me with your experiences you are having and the way you could put in words the effect your circumstances have on people around you and Bill. I also felt so understood in what I was trying to express in the piece on my blog on humanness. You have dealt with so much, for lack of a better way of putting it. I felt with you the pain and loneliness that have affected you as you are facing so much, so fast. I am so inspired by the faith you have and the way you view life in God's economy.

I could so appreciate the point you made about those who follow and are guided, in a sense, by our reaction and treatment of our life condition. I identified with you when you said some are removing themselves and are more comfortable with the safety of a greeting card. I concur and like you, I understand the fear and confusion people feel.

I have been doing better in the last few weeks than ever in the two years since I first went to complain of my tremors that started, seemingly out of the blue. I have gone through such a range of emotion, disappointment, fear, disbelief, curiosity, and on the list goes. Essentially, I was devastated and sinking inside my soul. I wrote a blog entry a few weeks ago about worship and how my body and mind don't always cooperate when I am trying to do what I love most, spend time in the house of God. I felt like I expressed it well and people were moved as they responded. Then, I wrote this more recent article about expressing our hurts and disappointments, citing Jesus as he faced the cross. Somewhere along the line, things began to click and I am getting much more feedback and many more readers are visiting.

While I was reading your reply, I reached a point where I put it all together in my mind and heart, realizing that I have passed through a very difficult period of adjustment to the depression and disappointment, to find myself back to being the Dan that I was since I decided to be a Christian so many years ago. I feel as though I can accept my disease and decline as being part of who I am, but I am able to see that God's love and deliverance is so powerful in my life and in the fabric of who he made me, that I am able to go on. I am not going on in my strength, but rather in the power of the cross and the resurrection.

I wanted to let you know that your responses to the blog and the discussion that ensued below both touched me deeply and helped me to galvanize my new learning and improved outlook. I am thinking of you and Bill, tonight and I can only offer my friendship and prayers for you both. I thank you for caring enough to write me such a thoughtful note and for the way you brought some things into clarity for me. How can I thank you, my friend, for your caring communication?

I wish you the peace of Christ. Take care, Dan

From Noreen

I THINK OTHER PEOPLE HAVE DIFFICULTY WITH "NO ANSWER OR SOLUTION". PERHAPS IT FRIGHTENS THEM. THEY WANT SOMETHING TO WORK: WE CAN SHOW THEM GOD. SHOWING THEM GOD IS NOT EASY, ESPECIALLY IF WE ARE AT A LOW POINT, BUT GOD WILL STREGTHEN US AND USE US. I THINK IT'S OK TO LET THEM SEE US "STRUGGLE." THAT'S WHEN GOD'S POWER SHOWS ITSELF....WHEN WE ARE WEAK, AND HE LIFTS US UP. IT ALSO GIVES OTHERS A CHANCE TO MINISTER TO US. SOME PEOPLE WILL BACK AWAY. I THINK THEY ARE AFRAID AND WONDER IF THEY COULD ENDURE THE PATH WE'RE WALKING.

THEY LOOK AT OUR SITUATIONS, AND SEE US "GOING ON," AS IN YOUR SONG, AND THEY WONDER. I BELIEVE THE LORD USES US AS EXAMPLES FOR THE BELIEVERS WALKING BEHIND US. THEY WATCH US AND HOPEFULLY ARE ENCOURAGED.

CHRISTIANS HAVE TOLD ME TO "KEEP MY CHIN UP! " AND YES, THAT WILL DO IT! I KNOW THEY THINK THAT IS ENCOURAGING. THEN THERE IS THE "SMILE," BUT FROM A DISTANCE.

I OPENLY ADMIT HOW DIFFICULT THIS IS, SO THEY PRAY FOR ME AND ASK ME WHAT TO DO. THERE ARE ONLY A FEW PEOPLE WHO WILL WALK RIGHT ALONG WITH ME THROUGH EVERYTHING.

AT THIS POINT IN OUR JOURNEY, I'M WATCHING SOME PEOPLE BACK AWAY. CARDS SEEM TO BE THE THING WITH WHICH THEY ARE MOST COMFORTABLE.

THE LORD IS BRINGING OTHER PEOPLE INTO OUR LIVES, THOUGH. HE PROVIDES.

REMEMBER, SOMETIMES THE LORD NEEDS TO GET US "ALONE" FOR AWHILE TO DEPEND ONLY ON HIM. THIS STRENGHTENS OUR FAITH IN HIM.

BILL AND I WILL SEE TARGET TODAY AND HAVE LUNCH.

GOD BLESS YOU FOR YOUR HONESTY AND TRANSPARENCY, DAN. NOREEN

More From Noreen

Dan, I'm afraid I didn't take time to answer one of your emails re: your blog, but I remember thinking that Jesus asked for His Father to take the cup from Him if it was possible. Does that fit your question? God made us, knows our emotions, and allows us to "feel" different things. We just need to be aware of depending on our feelings. There is a vast difference between – just "feeling"—rather than "believing by faith."

Blessings, Noreen

P.S. How are you and Karrie doing? Hope I spelled your "Karrie" correctly.

My Response to Noreen

Yes, you did actually spell her name correctly and I commend you, since that happens rarely.

Noreen, you are right. I appreciate your point about giving in to feelings, which may in turn produce doubt or fear, rather than faith. I think I would express these concerns only in the context of honesty before God. It seems sometimes people want to hear me answer, "Fine, the medications are doing wonders!" I know you can see the truth *as well as the humor* in this description. What I was trying to do was teach those of us dealing with neurodegenerative diseases, as the patient or close family member, to encourage an honest discussion and questions in order to strengthen our faith through the healing of questions. God brought Jesus through from that moment in the garden and raised him up as a victory over the power of darkness.

Thank you for your feedback. You have many friends to keep up to date. I keep you in prayer. Take care, Dan

Another Response to Noreen

Bill and Noreen, I appreciated seeing a photo of you and Bill on an outing. I am so happy for you both. It warms my heart to see this. Thank you, Dan

Author's Note: Noreen's beloved husband Bill passed away from complications of Multiple Systems Atrophy not long after this exchange.

Another Reader

Dear Dan,

I am so pleased to have come across your blog. My son-in-law also suffers with Parkinson's Plus– the MSA version. He started having symptoms in 2005 at the age of 42, and after a year of doctors and every test imaginable he was diagnosed with MSA. He was a youth pastor, but like you, he had to give up his work and succumb to this disabling disease. I have written to him about finding your blog, and have given him the web page so he can read it himself. I have told him about your music, and that I would like to order the CD for him. Please contact me or send the order form.

Thank You,
Marilyn

My Response to Marylin

Thank you Marylin, for your wonderful note. In spite of the condition that I have, I am just thrilled to be able to support and encourage others in facing this situation with faith in God. It is always a special moment each and every time I receive a message such as yours. I have attached the order form for my album. I pray that God will use my humble efforts to support my fellow Parkinson's Plus sufferers.

Please let your son-in-law know that he is welcome to contact me at any time. I am sure that I can learn from him, as well. I must say, it is significant when a man or woman in their prime, such as your son-in-law, develops such a serious illness. His ministry is something I am sure is hard to let go of, as was my career God called me to in the public schools. I feel for him! Please stay in touch. Again, I can't thank you enough for your email. God bless you today.
Dan

Chapter Six

With Faith I Will Go On

N THIS CHAPTER I have adapted individual articles written for the "PD Plus Me" online blog for the purpose of this book. Each one is an individual topic, and stands alone as a complete concept within the chapter as a whole. This chapter will focus on specific issues concerning how faith has had a major role in my accepting and living with a Parkinson's Plus condition.

God Understands Our Humanness

It happens without planning, without real awareness of those around us or the realization that we are doing anything intentionally. We have illness in our lives, some kind of chronic, or terminal, or persistently dangerous disease that many have in various ways, and we want to gloss over it. It isn't that we actually want to, but it is as though we are expected to do so. We have the impression that being a believer in God, a person of deep faith and conviction, means we don't have real human feelings or hurt, or loss, or anger, or disillusionment. But we do—let's be honest with ourselves! And you don't have to be seriously ill to feel these things. It may be the death of a close relative or friend, or a deep valley that started when you lost your job, your home, or yourself respect. It happens to all of us. We need to learn to express these things.

I sometimes get the impression that it is sinning against God to admit to a feeling of loneliness in the midst of depression, or to share concerns about fear of a shortened life or a difficult prognosis. We want to always present the image of a believer who knows that since God has given us eternal life, and a promise of His constant presence as being ever so real, that it ought to make dim all thoughts of accepting human suffering or feelings of insecurity. I don't think God the Father is asking that of us. I think He wants us to be real, as He does know our thoughts and the things we are facing are ever before Him, so we need not be ashamed to say that it hurts. Cry out to God! Let Him see your tears. Be real with yourself and Him. This is to be truly human and that is something beautiful in His sight.

We look into the life of Christ and see something more real, more passionate, more painful yet, that anything I am describing. And Jesus doesn't gloss over the pain and loneliness. In the Garden of Gethsemane He cries out to the Father to "Take this cup from me," and asks while on the cross the timeless utterance, "My God, my God, why has Thou forsaken me?"

What is really remarkable is that these expressions are powerful moments and phrases that may bring us to a special closeness with Him. They represent a deep honesty between the believer and the God of Heaven and Earth. They signify a deep desire to embrace all of life– the life in eternity, and the life God has so blessed us with on this earth. God's human creation and the biological environment He forged with His hands, His breath, His words, His heart, are truly miracles and things to behold. I wouldn't want to miss them, really. Why would I?

Let's not jump too far ahead of ourselves. Why not be real in the moment? When the emptiness strikes, learn from Jesus.

Consider how He expressed those deep emotions and waited for the answer. In His case, it didn't come in the form He was requesting. But He went on. He faced the struggle; the greatest challenge any individual ever faced in the history of human existence. There were great and important eternal purposes found in His going through with the very experience, in His humanness, He wanted to avoid. He was willing, of course, because after His request, He adds, "Not my will, but Thine be done." He said this as drops of real blood were sweating from His brow. In His suffering, He expressed His humanness, fully. He embraced the calling. He didn't gloss over the experience, but He accepted it willingly. He went through it, alone.

We too, can learn from Christ. It is important to express our honest fears, hopes for deliverance, feelings of being alone and even forsaken. That is where God meets us. In our honestly expressed doubts, questions, feelings of neglect, anger or separation. And yet, we do have an amazing faith in an amazing God, who has promised us forever. We don't dim that truth when we allow ourselves to talk about the pain. I don't intend to dwell on these subjects, nor do I in actuality. But let us allow those around us who are in these dark places to say what is on their minds and hearts, and let that moment have its purpose, too.

The chance to hear someone express what it feels like to be human in such a rare and, in a sense, beautiful way, will enlighten and teach. Then, we too can learn to say, "Not my will, but Thine be done." I don't want Parkinson's Plus, and sometimes it makes me angry or fearful or yes, even depressed. Expressing that brings me closer to others, and to God. It is then that He reminds me of the amazing deliverance He promised. Jesus had to go to Calvary's Hill, but it was God the Father who raised Him up on the third day. God will do the same for each of us. But that doesn't mean He is asking us to skip the human part.

He gave that to us, too. Each day brings something new and beautiful, if we are looking for it.

God is Our Refuge

During a meeting with my Pastor, he spoke to me about the refuge of God that is available to us at all times. He referred me to Psalms, chapter 71 and explained the meaning of refuge. First of all, God's children are refugees in need of refuge, which is defined as shelter, protection and comfort. God is all of these things for us. He is our refuge.

A year or so ago, I was in my yard enjoying the beautiful green and various spring colors of flowers my wife tends in the gardens. As I scanned the surroundings and marveled at the serenity, I spotted another example of refuge. Karrie has several birdhouses, as she has a hobby of collecting and creating them, artistically. There were two bird dwellings that I took great interest in on this particular morning. One was a traditional birdhouse, made of wood and pine cones, materials she found in the forest near the cabin of our dear friends. Karrie built this house and hung it on a shady tree in our backyard. I watched carefully as a mother bird flew up and poked a beak in the circular opening at the front of the house. In this refuge, baby birds were stirring and responding as mother met their every expectation and provided them with sustenance she had found in the surrounding ecosystem. These birds were safely tucked inside this refuge and were being sheltered, fed and protected.

To the right of this hand-built bird home, was another in the form of a nest. This was the tiniest little teacup of a nest, made of primarily light colored cloth and bits of tree twigs and grass. It was so small I almost missed it! Nearly instantaneously, another mother bird arrived to land and sit upon what surely were very tiny eggs. This bird was a hummingbird and it was the ultimate picture of both fragility and courage, a dichotomy, I admit. This mother bird was dark in color, with a long, thin, black beak, and as I watched her, I realized it was one of the few times I had ever seen a hummingbird in a still moment. She was not busily moving as it typically would do, not hovering in one place as wings flapped so fast they created a blur to the human eye. This mother was confidently and nobly sitting atop the nest, seemingly warming and protecting her most prized possession and heartfelt responsibility.

This hummingbird refuge struck me in two ways that are relevant to us, those who are forced to deal with serious illness. First, the nest was precariously clinging to a thin twig that drooped loosely from a larger branch above. It was there that this mother hummingbird had lovingly and painstakingly wrapped and weaved the construction materials as tightly and securely as possible to this branch, only slightly hidden behind large, green leaves. Unknown to the mother and the incubating chicks was the reality that this refuge, of dainty perfection, was completely dependent on the grace of this limp stick to maintain the safety of this diminutive family. And yet there it hung, suspended in time and in complete trust that an enemy, such as the masters of the property, would not come and accidentally bump, or even unknowingly slap, this miniature structure from its perch.

Secondly, this reminded me of the "refuge story" and the explanation I receive from my friend, Pastor Brad. He spoke of a placid harbor in a cove near an island that brought relief from a tempest sea he had experienced on a boating excursion. This natural calm area of the ocean came at just the right moment and provided a poignant example of the God of refuge spoken of in Psalm 71: 1-3.

"In you, O Lord, I have taken refuge; let me never be put to shame. Rescue me and deliver me in your righteousness;

turn your ear to me and save me. Be my rock of refuge, to which I can always go; give the command to save me, for you are my rock and my fortress." – The Holy Bible, New International Version

God understands the challenge brought by this illness, and the troubles many of you are facing right now resulting from other difficulties. He provides refuge, not as an escape, or even a permanent solution, to the perils of illness. He is with us to sustain us, guide us, give us strength and purpose, and to shelter us from the outside influences that will batter our ship as it sails through such a storm. Are there dangers or threats of physical loss, or even pain? Yes, and yet, through it all, God provides refuge.

Seeing these faithful and trusting mother birds, providing for their young, ready to face whatever strong wind or predator that would come, triggered my memory of the refuge story my Pastor had shared. These mother birds were secure in their confidence that everything would be all right. We, like the baby birds, are unaware of the perils that we face around the corner, but we can choose to trust the God of refuge who is faithful to provide the shelter, protection and guiding hand that we need. We too hang precariously from a flimsy human existence at times, but He has a harbor just around the bend if we will keep sailing on in our simple, child-like faith.

Brain Image and Parkinson's Plus

So now what? I find that I have MRI pictures of my brain that show atrophy in some vital areas that affect important life functions. Well, how do I respond to that news? I have come to the realization that I don't really have control in this situation. I spent my life with the belief that by taking responsibility for the outcomes in my life, I could make almost anything happen that I believed was important to me. I set out to walk in faith and follow God's steps as I set goals, chose a career, led my family and prioritized the things that were most important for my loved ones.

This Parkinson's Plus has written a different story about my life. It has taken my power to determine how my life will turn out. It isn't that I don't understand or can't accept that reality, it is that I am not familiar with how to go forward without the sense of personal responsibility or determination over my own fate that I have employed throughout my life. Anything, faced with faith in God, can be dealt with, overcome, accomplished or reached with the right outlook and an unselfish purpose. At this point, I have to learn a whole new meaning of helplessness.

This is total surrender—humility at its core. I wonder how to make the most of the life I have? I only know how to do what I have always done—trust God and think of every difficulty as an opportunity. I will make this into something good, somehow. That is all I know. I refuse to give in to despair and futility. Not with my wonderful wife at my side seeing me through this. Not with the greatest kids any dad ever had to inspire me and to lift my spirits. I am sticking this thing out, no matter what.

Families Facing Fears Together- Drawing Close

I am more and more aware as time passes that this Parkinson's Plus disease is real. Let me explain. The first year was a whirlwind of learning, almost standing back in an objective posture and reading everything I could find to make sense of what the doctor's were telling me and what I was experiencing. The second year brought a lot of sadness and puzzlement, and at times deep depression, as I attempted to figure out why this was happening to my family and me. It was two years ago that I first went to a doctor to ask what was causing a tremor that was in my head, neck, hands and legs. There was much to do in these first two years, and the grieving cycle was certainly a big part of that period.

The third year is underway and there are some discoveries involved. I have become more comfortable with the reality of what has happened and continues to happen as this disease progresses. In the first year it was frightening, yes, but in some ways it was a curiosity that I could investigate and research. That's what I do. I read and write about things I am experiencing. That is what my career was about, so I saw no reason to not carry on with that same approach. As time went along, and the diagnosis was determined, the seriousness of the disease began to really hit me and take me down, along with my family. Each of us has a process of grieving and acceptance to undergo. It doesn't happen in the same manner in each case, because each person's life is being affected differently. Simple platitudes of "God must have a reason" and "God only chooses special people to give serious illness" (as though a neurological disease is a privilege) don't really relieve any of the stress on our adult children or my wife. Those are things that a family member needs to realize as they experience the fears, threats, hopes, let downs and realities for themselves. This is something I am becoming more and more aware of as I am around my family members, whom I love so much it hurts. It hurts to know what they have to face. There are just no easy answers.

Today, as I am in the start of a third year, I am beginning to realize for myself that this Parkinson's Plus condition is part of who I am. I guess you will understand what I mean when I say that it always was going to become a part of me and I embrace it, in that sense. The fact that it has robbed me of abilities and dreams, to one degree or another, isn't an easy thing to embrace by any means, but the realization that I can make the best of each day I have, is a thought born out of those losses.

I have the gift of knowing that each day is precious and the beauty of the people in my life, family and friends, are the wonders I focus upon. The many years I spent planning for the next career advancement, studying for graduate and postgraduate degrees to make myself more competitive in seeking positions in education, was a way of life. I loved the struggle to come out on top! I must add, though, that my career was always about the kids and adults I wanted to lead and be there for—to teach and encourage. But the focus on where to live, where to work, how much to earn and what title I felt suited me was a distraction from living *today*. Living in the now is a great thing to learn to do. I am sorry it took a serious, life threatening disease to help me achieve that, but I am grateful nonetheless.

I don't need someone else to tell me what I should learn from this circumstance, I have to find that truth for myself. Hearing it just doesn't make the same impact. My beautiful treasures of grown children, and my loving wife, have these things to go through on their own, with my support. I think what I have learned from them is the respect they each need and deserve as they face this illness, as individuals. We are a close and loving family. We don't take suffering in our family lightly, nor does any family that has its priorities in order. I regret that they have to deal with these things because of some exposure to chemicals, a head trauma or some other factor that I came in contact with that brought me to this place of neurological loss and decline. There is also the strong possibility that it is just a defect in my own physical makeup.

I am choosing life and the things I can do—to sing and play my guitar, to read, to converse, and beyond all that, *to be with my very dear and special family*. They waited a long time for me to be home—I am going to appreciate it.

Two "Dans" No Longer

In another of the many moments that I have thought about the way this condition was affecting my life, I decided to take stock. I have adjusted and accepted my neurological condition to a point, no question. I have gone through the initial two years of grief and loss, along with the realization that life will never be the same.

I have been able to get past the depression of finding that I have this illness and I worked at being up and having purpose for my life. In spite of everything, I have a wonderful family life, with a loving and supportive family. No man could be more blessed. I have been given ministries to others through the internet and also in my music. With all of these things to fulfill me, what is the question that remains unanswered, then?

I have begun to realize that what once was an objective reality, the onset of this disease, has become more and more real to me, as the one it is affecting. Originally, it was as though I was still me, but I was watching someone else, named, "Dan," go through these incredible medical challenges. Let me explain this in more detail.

I have the physical situation, where my disabilities are growing gradually, insidiously, like a green blob invading my life. It creeps and creeps, relentlessly attacking my nerves, muscles, fingers, feet, legs, mouth, face, eyes, neck and spine. Every part of me is being affected. Walking with any coordination is becoming more and more difficult. It is just a matter of time before I start spending more time in a wheelchair, and I am fighting it with all my might. The times I need it most are those involving a long distance from the car to the event, or a store that requires a lot of walking such as a Costco or Target. Also, if a lot of time standing to visit is required in a given situation, I have to have a place to sit so that I won't have to hold myself up as my body shakes and twists. Sometimes it is the pain in my feet and lower legs that forces me to go find a place to sit. The involuntary swaying of my legs and spine make balance and staying on my feet more difficult.

More than anything, I can tell my mind is slipping a bit, but ever so gradually. As you've read in previous chapters in this book, or have looked further into Parkinson's or Parkinson's Plus, you know that cognitive complications are expected. For example, Progressive Supranuclear Palsy and Corticobasal Ganglionic Degeneration are both caused by taupathies in the brain tissue, and in some cases, may have a relationship with Fronto-temporal Dementia (FTD). This is not to say that I have FTD, just that I am aware of the possibility, and thus I am mentioning it here as an honest apprehension.

I hurt my neck in an auto accident in the fall of 2007, and when I found out that it is a four-disc injury, I realized that this was an additional dilemma added to my Parkinson's Plus. PD Plus has already caused Dystonia (stiffness, twisting, or jerking) of my neck and back. My neck twists forward and down, or sometimes turns up and arches back, depending on my posture and what I am doing. The neck tremor, bobbing/nodding, is occurring while my discs are bulging and it just increases the pain. I have a hard time imagining my life in the future with this spine and neck pain, all the while with my neck twisting and jerking. It seems like a very bad situation as my life goes on and I face this reality with faith that God will see me through.

I know that the way I am and the way I have changed, with the losses and disabilities, have caused some confusion. I am in a very strange world inwardly, and it seems I will never be able to truly explain this perception to another person in a way that it is understandable. I don't think there are words in the English language that would help me describe what it is like to have a disease that threatens to take my ability to move, speak, swallow, breath or think. I try not to dwell on it, and have been pretty successful at doing this, but I am not able to ignore it too well anymore. For the first seven months, I honestly thought that I was experiencing the onset of a fast progressing case of Parkinson's, but that wasn't to be. As difficult as Parkinson's is, it is a more gradually progressing condition, and individuals have been known to remain active in professional life and physical hobbies for a number of years. I had to get the version that is "like PD on Steroids" (as one of my dear friends once coined)!

I am trying to look forward to some wonderful days with the abilities I have right now. My attitude is good, but I am truly scared. I have a healthy fear, but I keep it in check most of the time, pretty well. Karrie knows about how this is affecting me, but I don't want her to worry any more than she does already.

Which brings me to the point I began with: I once viewed this whole process as though it was happening to a person outside of me. It was as though I was two men—one who was the old Dan who was a husband, father, educator, high achiever, musician, clown who loved to make others laugh, and sports enthusiast. Then there was the other Dan, the man with the neuro-degenerative disease. I thought of that second man as an objective reality – someone outside of myself. This is how a situation like this really affects you.

I read with interest the information about Parkinsonism and diseases that result from neuronal loss and how they progress. I studied hard on the symptoms and the resulting difficulties. Then, around the 18-month mark, which was in April of 2007, I began to see how this objective other man, with a degenerative disease, was merging with the man I am. It became clearer and clearer to me that I was that second man. In recent weeks, I think I have crossed that divide completely and recognized that I am one man, no longer a dichotomy. The diseased brain of the other, objective man, who went through a differential diagnostic process with one of the best neurologists in the area, was actually me—the Dan I have always been and always will be. We have merged and I now know what it is that is happening to me. That second Dan, with the condition, doesn't now eclipse the first, but we have blended and now are clearly "one" in my perception. Now, I can fight this disease as it is happening to me, not just the objective other man that I used to find so interesting to study. No, Parkinson's Plus is my disease and it is part of who I am, the life I live and it has been injected into everything about me.

I am not giving in to fear or quitting, I am just recognizing the place I am in and working toward a determination to make the very most of everything I still have. No one is more supported, loved or blessed by family and friends that surround me. I thank each and every one of you for your love and prayers. I don't have all the answers right now. I am going to keep growing—we all are, if we choose to do so. I simply had this realization, and since I know that I am one man now (I mean this figuratively, of course), that tells me that somehow this neuro-degenerative disease has always been a part of the Dan I am.

God knows the Dan that is the man I have always been, and the one whose life has manifested this growing medical crisis. The first step in real growth is acceptance and recognition of the truth. The truth is no longer evasive; it has become too visible for me to ignore. I have become "one" and God has been there all along the way. *He embraced me, with this disease, before I realized what was happening.* Somehow that gives me a strong sense that "His plans are not my plans, and His ways are not my ways." We will go forward, with Him leading us through every mountaintop and valley experience. Both are bound to appear on my horizon.

When Life Throws you a Curve

It hit me like a fastball in the late innings. I was angry that this disease had come into my life, but I thought I had dealt with that a year or two ago, and that we had moved to the next phase: getting on with life and making the most of the beautiful things we have in family, friends, and the many blessings we are fortunate to experience. I forgot something a dear friend told me not long ago. Exactly how he said it, I am not sure. But this wise friend said something similar to the following paraphrase:

"The grief process is cyclical, not linear."

Things we think we have worked out circle back to trouble us and we go through the anger, denial, acceptance, and healing all over again. Disease, or loss of any kind, bring a grief process that is more than a mere diagram. You may choose not to process the grief and try to ignore it. It isn't a paradigm you choose—grief happens and you go through it willingly or otherwise.

I have chosen to grapple with it, but in my humanness, I sometimes forget that my own strength isn't going to be enough. For me, I need Christ's strength that doesn't have limits and His love that has no boundaries. He will go where I am; He meets me in this place of anger, fear, frustration, loneliness or bitterness. He brings the rain of peace, and it washes over you, sometimes when you least expect it.

I have been feeling sorry for myself, again, and feeling critical and defensive. It goes something like this. "Who really understands what I am facing? No one can share these inward experiences that I have as a result of the neurological problems I have to deal with, day in and day out." Then, a close friend named Orville got my attention and reminded me that it is no one's fault. God hasn't abandoned me or my family. To the contrary He is there with me, right in the midst of the chaos. Here is a bit of what Orville wrote to me, as a way of helping me understand what it is like to be on the outside looking in and wanting to do something—anything to help.

"I do not understand life, even though at times I think I do. A hard breaking curve has been thrown at you, but you are still at the plate preparing for the next pitch. Your strength is evident. I wish I could take a pitch for you, but I can't and I know you would not want me to."

Because my friend and I were both athletes in our younger years, and we still fancy ourselves as such, this metaphor really made sense to me and opened my mind to the truth. I am supposed to take the pitch myself, even if it is up and in, right at the helmet. I have always been one to get back in the batters box and get ready to hit the next one, hard. My friend was right. I can do this, but I can't do it in my own strength.

Why does it take an experience such as a neuro-degenerative disease for us to learn and relearn the lessons we received so many years before?

Come on. Bring the heat—the high, fast one. I am ready.

More on the Journey

An Atypical Parkinsonism condition like the one I have affects a person in a variety of ways, and like any disease, there are up days and down days. Recently, I am having a particular difficulty with feeling weakness all over, and it is most noticeable in my hands and arms. I went with Karrie to the grocery store where I always take my scooter and get items Karrie sends me for on her list. The best I could do on this occasion was to follow her from aisle to aisle. Also, I bag the groceries from my scooter at the end of our shopping. Helping with the grocery shopping is a great outing for me and is also something I can do to help my wife and sons.

During this outing, due to the weakness, it was tough to fill the bags and lift them over the edge to place them in the cart. My arms were exhausted when I finished bagging half of the food and placing it in the cart. While shopping I had trouble keeping my body from slumping down in the scooter, and my hands were in awkward positions as I tried to grip the handles that I use to steer the scooter. On top of this, I was struggling to avoid the eye crossing and double images that kept occurring, and is a frequent condition, meaning it happens daily to one degree or another. Finally, my head and neck tremor, which is persistent, was making it harder to use the scooter and sit comfortably. This head tremor, which involves my torso as well, is known as "titubation."

It was during this same week that I noticed it was hard to speak on the phone with my father and he was having trouble hearing me, since my voice was softer than at other times and I tend to murmur. This occurs because my mouth and tongue don't move properly and with normal coordination. This too is an expected symptomatic aspect of atypical Parkinsonism, disorders which include Parkinson's Plus syndromes.

I felt a tough period coming on yesterday when it was a struggle to walk around the house with coordination and normal strength. It makes it doubly hard because I have a lot of joint pain all over, but particularly in my neck and lower back. The nerves in my lower back are being compressed from years of back injuries and three back surgeries, so this leads to severe sciatic pain.

In spite of these struggles I am hopeful and full of joy. God is strengthening my heart and spirit through these challenges and I am going on in faith. As I said yesterday, I know that, "I can do everything through Him who gives me strength." (Philippians 4:13). I have too much to appreciate in light of our loving family and friends to let these things get me down. Life is beautiful and every good thing we experience is a gift.

My Internal World

Sitting here, reviewing the day, I realize that once again I am struggling with the thought of those I have known and cherished as friends and colleagues seeing me in a different form. I have been a friend, boss, leader, fellow musician, and colleague to some great people over the years. I want to be the same friend and companion I would have been in the past, but it is not possible.

How do I explain that I don't care any less, but that I don't want to be viewed the way I have become—slower to speak, less clear, and with fewer expressions? I want to choose to participate in activities and events, but I stop myself when I perceive the potential of altering the way I will be remembered by those I once worked along side, or led as a manager. I want to be involved to the extent that I can, considering how my energy gives out in a short two-hour period, but I want to be able to be the person outwardly I know is still inside.

Being in a wheelchair at locations that require long periods of standing or longer distances walking, is an absolute necessity now, but it too, at times, keeps me home. I don't mind the shaking really, as I have explained in my recent blog entry. I expect that it will be noticeable at times, and at others, not so much. Sometimes the hardest day to be with others is when I have a constant internal tremor disrupting my ability to sit or stand comfortably, but it looks like I am having a great day. When, oh when, will this eternal shaking stop?

Sometimes I am conversing and really enjoying myself, and the other person turns double in my visual field. I have heard many a great sermon in church staring through the distraction of my eyes crossing as a result of the part of my brain that governs eye movements malfunctioning. And what a headache this causes as it strains my eye muscles!

I notice little things. Today, a "Monday," I referred to as "Friday" while enjoying a drive with a dear friend. It felt like I had no idea where I was in space. I was disoriented in relation to recent occurrences. This is a frequent experience for me. It isn't as though I didn't get up in the morning and read the paper, watch the news on CNN, and become aware of the calendar. It is two hours later, and I had lost track of it all. I do not like that feeling. How many times have I forgotten where Karrie took me in the minivan twenty minutes before? Enough times to know the changes in my mind are concrete and hard to easily accept.

It seems that when I try to explain how I feel it is like I am building a block wall around myself. The more I attempt to explain what it is like to have a neuro-degenerative disease, the more I find myself thinking, "Why bother explaining this?" I am not discontent, or unsettled or down. I am simply seeing these issues for what they are—it is not easy to share the effects of this disease with people to much of any depth, at all. I can express myself well on the computer, but there are neurological issues that keep my speaking process from occurring the way it once did, so naturally.

Somewhere, down deep, I have the answers and the descriptive language to write here what this loneliness feels like. I am comfortable at home because my dear ones are accustomed to who I am and what I fight. At the same time, I think they remember the father and husband I was before brain cells began to be affected. I don't feel confident about that with those outside of the home as easily, and it isn't about anything that they are doing or saying.

It is that I see a reflection of myself in their eyes, on their faces. My smile used to be contagious and would elicit smiles from others. I recognize the blankness that my friends and extended family are experiencing on my face as it is mirrored in their expression. Their smiles, given in the face of what is a frown on my end, are a gift like no other. I have seen those hopeful expressions many times, and wondered where each beautiful individual finds a smile while gazing into the emptiness I am projecting toward them, so unintentionally.

I retreat to my computer world, where there are new friends who in reality I have never seen in person or even heard their voices. I am able to know them easily, as those who have been where I am going, with their husband, mother or wife, who has lost the fight to PSP or MSA in previous months or years. Some of my recent online friends are patients and able to share the experiences with me. Still others are in the middle of doing what Karrie does—care giving for their loved one. This gets me through the day and provides a no-explanation-needed interaction, where they have seen similar problems and struggles that I regularly encounter.

I am used to being the one people depend on. In the world outside of my family and friends, I was accustomed to being an educational leader, an active musician, and a part time graduate school instructor. These things are all compromised, but who I am, in essence, lives on. My heart still beats to the sound of great acoustic, gospel, R and B, country and rock 'n roll music. I still track every swing and every pitch of the LA Dodgers. I passionately follow the Lakers and dream of another world championship.

My family is still my strongest passion, and Karrie my greatest love. I can read CS Lewis, Phillip Yancy, Howard Zinn and Frank Peretti. I regularly break out one of my guitars and drift off as I sing a song of worship or a love song I cherish from the past. At times, my fingers fumble in a way they never did, with the exception of my days as a seven and eight-year-old boy learning my first songs. I admit a great disappointment When

I miss something on a guitar fret or string, which would have been as sure as the sun rising in the east in my strong grip in days past. After this abnormal movement disorder took residence in my body, abilities I once took for granted became unreliable.

I didn't drive today. That is not new; I haven't driven since February of 2006. But everyday, I want to pick up the keys and grab the wheel. On bad days, I dream of a new Toyota truck or that Corvette I never drove. This, too, I accept. It isn't necessary to drive to call yourself a man.

I must confess, it is often nice to sit back and watch scenery I never noticed before as Karrie drives wherever we go. The good news is she is much better than I was at paying attention to the road and not talking while driving!

I will be content to live the life I have with the gifts few can claim—a wonderful marriage with years of happiness behind and more ahead to cherish. Add four great adult kids that are talented, caring people, successful human beings and solid citizens, and you have a doubly blessed man. Above all, I have faith in a living and loving Savior who promises to be with us through it all. He covers us in His wings and holds us in the hollow of His hand.

I won't gloss over the everyday, the empty times, and the loneliness that can be pervasive. I am not giving in to it, rather I am looking it in the face as Daniel looked the lion in the mouth in his den.

Writing these thoughts down gives me a better understanding. Now, if I can just explain this verbally, the next time I have the privilege of sitting and visiting with one of my good friends.

Keep on Singing - or Do What You Love

I would like to begin by giving a report on how things went with regard to playing and singing with my son, Mark and another musician friend on Sunday morning. It went well, as I led worship, played and sang for our church's contemporary service. It was a privilege to serve in this way, and I must say, with reference to the subject of this blog, it was physically very challenging. In spite of the facts—that I had to be seated throughout, that it was tough getting up to the stage, and that my eyes had difficulty tracking the music charts I arranged to lead the band—it was a wonderful experience.

One of the most cherished things that I consider a central, critical part of life is the opportunity to sing Christian music in my home church. I wrote my first gospel song in 1972, and I have sung in churches, coffee houses, camps, schools, auditoriums, banquet rooms and in TV and radio studios since that time. The difference is that I no longer am able to take for granted that I will be able to pull off the event with ease, physically. Knowing that I can't be sure my hands and voice will work when I call on them, makes it a matter of faith as I walk up on the stage and take my seat. So on this occasion, when I tucked my 1976 Guild D55 acoustic guitar under my arm and pulled my chair up to the microphone, I felt that familiar stirring of energy and excitement in my chest. I glanced over my shoulder to see my son, Mark, sticks in hand and on his stool, ready for the downbeat on his drum kit. Having my son along side me, brought back that old familiar feeling of pure musical joy I have grown to love since I played my first concert at the age of 17 in Lakewood, California.

The uniqueness now, is that because I treasure so much my abilities to sing and play, I am moved that I have this one more chance to do what I love—to sing my heart out for God and for the people assembled in His House. It has become a fulfillment of purpose and reminds me that my life goes on, though I am diagnosed with Parkinson's Plus. I appreciate Pastor Brad's openness and willingness to give me these opportunities and it is so inspiring to have that support. Each and every time I lead or perform, I cherish the experience, as it technically could be my last.

I know that it is probable that at some point, the little mistakes on the guitar, forgotten lyrics, or unwanted movements will add up to a choice not to put my less-than-best performance out on the stage. I want to "go out" (i.e., stop performing) knowing that I still am able to prepare and give my best, and I don't want to change the way my music is remembered by those for whom I love to sing. This is an issue that has many facets, and I don't claim to have my views all figured out in this regard. For now, I am so thankful for my Pastor and fellow members/attendees, as they are more than generous with their support.

Secondly, Karrie, Stephen and I continue to get treatment for our neck and back strains. Of late, they are progressing in a fair manner, but there are still issues of limitations on movement for both Karrie and Stephen, and some considerable pain in Karrie's case. I am presently having very severe neck and upper back pain, and my neck stiffness is very limiting. I have been resting and staying at home the last two days, hoping to see improvement. As recently as yesterday, the pain was not improving and is still making the movement of my head and left arm very difficult.

It occurs to me that Progressive Supranuclear Palsy, which is the Parkinson's Plus condition I have been told is likely to be my diagnosis, involves a very stiff or rigid neck and spine. The accident may have hastened this condition, although I am still hoping to improve soon. Another name for PSP is "Nuchal Dystonia Dementia Syndrome," which one should note, includes the word, "Dystonia."

Dystonia is the condition causing cramping and stiffness of muscles and joints, along with the problems of twisting, repetitive movements that affect the neck, torso, limbs, eyes, face, vocal chords, and/or a combination of these affected neuro-muscle functions. Dystonia isn't about muscle or joint dysfunc-tion, but rather a problem that originates in the movement center of the brain. It can't be fixed mechanically, but must be treated medically.

Listed below is an excellent internet site that describes some Parkinson's Plus conditions very well and has some unique ex-planations that are worth reading.

http://medicine.jrank.org/pages/1196/Multiple-System-Atro-phy.html

Can God Redeem Any Circumstance?

The phrase "God can redeem any circumstance" is something you may have heard on broadcasts, read in books or heard quoted from the lectern. I heard it repeated in recent months and it jumped into the pages of the narrative of my life in the years since being diagnosed with a movement disorder. I think that this is a very important thought to consider. When faced with Parkinson's Plus syndrome, Parkinson's Disease, or the struggles and foibles of our human existence, what does such a phrase suggest? Does it imply that a cure, a miracle healing, a door out of a situation into a world where pain and difficulty are always fixable is always around the corner? Or does it stand for something else more concrete, more substantial that you can truly count on no matter what?

The latter of the two options is, at least for me, the best interpretation. With the risk of sounding like I am oversimplify-ing the answer to this question, God can redeem any struggle, serious ailment, loss of employment or serious family problem. We don't know how God will work in a given circumstance, but we should feel the freedom to ask God to heal a body, bring us the financial help we need or cause a fractured marriage to be restored with immediacy. Certainly God is able to miraculously bring the solution to any overwhelming difficulty, but ultimately we ask knowing that He will carry out His sovereign will.

What we can count on is God's presence in our lives and His never ending love to carry us through life's biggest valleys. He is willing to walk us through a process of facing the initial, if not long lasting, grief or loss process. He is there to give us strength and, if necessary, to carry us in His arms as we lay our burdens on Him through our simplest prayers.

He is our teacher and our guide as we address the concrete needs that arise in the darkest of times. He seems to bring people into our path to befriend us, to comfort us and to be His hands, His feet and His voice ringing out in our dark night. He will speak to us through His "still small voice" to bring reassurance of His constant care that does not have limits.

God can redeem any difficulty or circumstance. We will go on being human and struggling, sometimes less and at times, incredibly, with a sense of "How could this be happening to me and my family?" God will meet us in the midst of the struggle and He will bring a contentment and joy that is unexplainable. It isn't always in the form of a miraculous solution or healing, but isn't His eternal love and redemption what we need most?

I will not attempt to diminish the pain and hurt you may be going through right now. I will not offer trite platitudes that some will parrot, even mockingly, as they point out alleged promises that we will always be healed, delivered, cash will arrive mysteriously in the mail, or our wandering teenage child will appear at our doorstep. To the contrary, problems are seemingly ours to solve as a part of the human condition, and yet God does walk beside us and love us unwaveringly as we grow and struggle through such trials.

God can redeem any circumstance. What we learn, how we grow and how we touch others lives in the midst of our greatest anguish, may be outcomes that we come to see as gifts from God. He gives us His Spirit, and the family and friends He puts in our path, to join us in the long journey. We too can reach out to others in similar circumstances and offer a hand as a brother, sister or friend.

Giving Thanks in All Circumstances

There are many times in our lives when we face circumstances that seem insurmountable, and yet we press on. This is not a linear process, as I have discussed in prior entries. The experience of struggling to accept, to face up to fears and to move on to a new day does not happen once and end there. We travel in a great circle, with a broadly sweeping journey, recognizing the crisis, grieving the loss of wellness or a loved one, pass through a time of anger, followed by disillusionment and finally acceptance. About the time we accept our altered life, something happens that reminds us of the reality of what has changed, and we find ourselves angry again. Sound familiar?

Presently, my journey has taken me through a number of plateaus and valleys along the way. I would define my present state of progress as being at a point of disillusionment growing into acceptance. How many times have I thought, "I have both feet on the ground and I accept the movement disorder affecting my mind, body and spirit?" Here I am again, in a place of accepting my situation. The good news for us all, is we do get to a place of peace, though in our humanness, it is not a permanent destination. It is more of a refueling station.

Acceptance doesn't mean being in a state of bliss, or necessarily, even happiness. But there is joy. Joy runs deeper and reminds us that our lives have purpose. For those who put their faith in God, He is our constant purpose, accompanying us all along our path, at each and every high or low point.

I don't believe God approves more of us when we reach the acceptance stage. Does that make sense for you, too? God loves us as much or more in the times of fear, frustration, anger and disillusionment. How do I know? I see His Son on the cross declaring that He is forsaken, and yet we know ultimately He was not. He rose triumphantly three days later from the tomb!

Lately, this acceptance has brought me to the renewed understanding of the blessings that accompany the struggle. My wonderful friend and sister, Teri, two years older than me, had her birthday in recent days. She has stood by me in heartfelt support through all of my life's exhilarating highs and deeply disappointing lows. What a lucky man I am to have a sister to be a friend and pal, when we as little ones drove our parents crazy with our antics, or when she accompanied me as a singer in my early days on stage. Now, as we have reached our midlife, Teri is a friend with which to grow old. Though miles separated us, our faith in God and the love of our family did not forsake us.

We are fortunate and blessed, but we have to look beyond the circumstances to realize that not everything in life goes our way. But look up and see that you are loved, you have friends, you have family and you have purpose. I am so thankful for the many wonderful friends I have that have supported my family and me, through the years. I deeply appreciate my parents, my brothers, my grandparents—who continually prayed for me through the years—and my own family. My sons are my pride and strength. No experience in my life equals their births and the privilege of raising such fine young men. My daughter-in-law is a gift that I thank God for often. My wife is my life and focus of all I do. How she saw something in me those 27 years ago, I will never know. I just realize how perfect she is for me, to complement me in my shortcomings and to be the one He intended for me. I wonder what I would have accomplished, without her giving me the encouragement and unselfish support that I needed to face those many challenges?

Though I express my appreciation today, I know that sometimes these blessings are obscured in our natural course of self-absorption. I know at times I have let people down when I was not always sure of why I had to face the movement disorder I fight and struggle with everyday. But even in my darkest nights I see you, my friends and family, shinning through as God's hands and voice, reassuring me of the blessings I have that remind me to be eternally thankful.

Progression Brings New Challenges

Where are we today with Parkinson's Plus? It is progressing, that much I know. Changes are both alarming, as well as subtle, in some cases, so it is not easy to give a quick summary of my health status. I have noticed that since the automobile accident, which strained my neck at impact when we were rear-ended, I have a jerkier, spastic walking gait. I feel more off balance and a certain degree of dizziness. When I walk, I meander along the side walk, never just walking the short distance between two points, which would be straight, presumably. Also, my head and neck tremor is more pronounced and it moves side-to-side and randomly switches to an up-and-down movement.

I do notice that my hands are a bit weaker in sensation. The practical implications are that I am having a bit of trouble with accuracy when I am playing the guitar and also, I have begun to drop things—examples are a drinking glass that crashed to the floor and a comb will fall from my hand as I begin to groom my hair. The pinkie finger on my left hand has always functioned as a single note "lead" while I am in a chord and singing one of my songs. I will miss my lead tones that I am used to playing in the background as I finger pick my chord behind my lyrics. Often, my fork slips from my grasp as I spastically try to catch it before it injures me or the individual with whom I am eating. I guess Karrie is at the greatest risk (forgive my sick attempt at humor)!

Cramping and pain in my lower legs, and particularly in my feet, is gradually increasing. My jaw tends to set and my teeth involuntarily clinch together, making singing harder to do freely. I am getting a slightly different tone out of my voice. I would describe my vocalization as being more strained sounding and somewhat nasal-like. Hey, it works for the great James Taylor, right? He made nasal vocal quality the standard for folk-rock guitarists!

I am forgetting things more, such as conversations I have had a week before. I will think I haven't heard from someone for a month or two, and I find out that we wrote each other an email in the last week. It is hard to stay organized when you forget what you were planning to do. I must be more disciplined about writing things down. I see strangers in stores and restaurants, and immediately feel sure I know them. It seems I am aware of this, but in my confusion, I seem to know everyone! The longer ago something happened, the better I remember it.

I am walking on in my life. This weekend, my son Mark, who is a drummer, guitarist, and vocalist, and I are starting a new CD. I have chosen 10 of my songs to record with a friend who has some great equipment and a college degree in sound production. We are very thankful to him for giving this a try, to see how we do on a few tracks. We will work primarily on percussion this week.

I am excited about three new songs I have written, and these will be added to songs I have written in previous years, and were not include on my first two CD's. One is a song written years ago by a friend I met in my high school youth group at church. I call it "Susie's Song" after the young lady who wrote it. Susie frequently reads my blog to the present day. I think this is a great collection of songs I have in mind for this project! Time will tell if I am able to sing well enough due to the effects of Parkinson's Plus, or if my hands will function effectively so I am able to get the quality performance I need. I will push through and work around the weaknesses in my voice and hands. With a positive attitude and a determined spirit, we will get this done. A long day of recording is physically difficult, if not mentally draining, literally.

I will be calling on talented friends and relatives to share their music skills with things like lead guitar parts, background vocals or electric bass. We are fortunate that the studio engineer is also a well-rounded musician. Between my son Mark's voice for harmonies, guitar ability and his expertise, drumming, we have a lot between the three of us to work with from the outset.

I will keep on doing the things I can do. I struggle with minor cognitive issues, but it is not just the brain fade jokingly called a "senior moment." It is so much more. Between my slowed cognition and struggles with speech, it is very frustrating at times. I would say that the severity we are talking about comes and goes. It is not a static issue, depending on the medication cycle and the rise and fall of the neurotransmitters in my brain. Though, I can no longer carry out my professional activities, I am able to share information for my support group, or provide music at our church. The blog site I write on the internet gives me a purpose and allows me to serve others, while making important connections.

There are many blessings and great opportunities in my life, in spite of the setbacks and disappointments. I really feel that overall, life is going well. My ability to accept the situation I am in and make the most of what I have, especially my wonderful family and faith in God, enables me to find myself joyful and full of gratitude.

What Does it Mean to Say: "I Will Go On?"

I am excited to share with you about how doors of opportunity are opening for me to be of service to others. A year before publishing this book, I began to think about giving up on writing it at all. I thought I would just fade into the shadows, to wallow in self pity over my progressive illness. Not long after, several people began to contact me online to let me know that my blog (interactive website) was helping them or a loved one dealing with Parkinson's or another neuro-degenerative disease. After those initial contacts, I began to see how I could continue to encourage others and provide information from a patient's perspective that is really making a difference. Putting it all in the context of faith was what brought it all into focus and provided the meaning for this book I began writing and designing in the form of a blog site in December 2006.

Next, I began to have opportunities to sing, keeping in mind that my ability to speak smoothly and perform at my normal level were both being demonstratively affected by Parkinson's Plus. To explain to you that I feel a limitation inwardly is to make a huge understatement. What is detectable is only a small fraction of what I feel when I am speaking, planning, or responding to questions. My hand coordination, especially with the finer dexterity needed to play a song to a perfected level, is gradually slipping from my control. Vocally, I am having difficulty with moving my mouth, as bradykinesia slows muscle movements throughout my body. The mouth, eye-lid, throat, tongue and facial muscles are no exception, thus my singing is moving toward a more nasal sound as I have less ability to use my voice dynamics. My higher pitches are limited a bit by the affect on my throat muscles. For now, I am able to compensate, and though I am not satisfied because of my perfectionist tendencies, these things are not very detectable by the audience at this point. My confidence that made getting on the stage a great drive since I was 11 years old and playing in my first garage band, is being shaken!

Every few months, God apparently chooses to use me, in spite of these things! I sing for our church's Sunday Seniors Luncheon as the guest performer and I really get excited about those opportunities. Also, I perform at events such as a hospice memorial for the families of those who have passed in the last year after bouts with serious illness. It is a privilege to sing for those who invite me to do so.

The local Parkinson's support group that Karrie and I belong to hosts a monthly meeting at a local church on the third Tuesday of the month. In the year prior to completing this book, I was invited to talk about Parkinson's Plus and follow up with the performance of some songs. When we share our interests and hobbies, we demonstrate the importance of staying active and not giving up. This reminds other patients and their caregivers that we need to preserve our abilities that are generated neurologically and thus subject to the effects of Parkinson's Plus or another movement disorder.

A married couple that is as dear as any Karrie and I have ever known had their 30th anniversary party in the last 12 months. I was asked to sing a special song for them, and again, this was an inspiration for me to keep going on.

I know that these things that I am being blessed with the opportunity to serve in are a gift to my spirit and a benefit to not only the audience, but to my family and me, as I struggle to remain as sharp as I am able to be. The cognitive aspects that are affected by my illness are the most difficult to overcome, in spite of the physical struggles I have in walking, controlling my eye movements and using my hands in a coordinated manner.

I am so thankful for those who have reached out to me to let me know I am helping them somehow by God's grace, and for others who have invited me to speak or sing at events. I am very motivated by these engagements.

The fact that I am not going to be as smooth a speaker as I was as an educational leader prior to my illness, and the fact that I may make errors that I have never been accustomed to as a musician in the past, is a reality that comes with these efforts. I was forced to retire because of my disabilities, but there are abilities that remain and that I need to maintain through such activities. True humility is a hard lesson and it takes a lifetime to learn!

I will continue to go on. There is so much to do and some things that are by God's design and how he made me—to sing, to teach and learn. This includes learning from those I have the privilege of getting to know in the process!

Faith Springs from Disillusionment

I want to preface what I am writing today with this thought. I have tried, as much as I felt appropriate, to be honest with myself and, in that sense, with you, in regards to the things I have written in this book. I have shared the times I have felt the blessings and closeness of God in my life. I have confessed to being human and having fear and doubts during the most troubling time of my life, after being diagnosed with a neuro-degenerative disease. However, I have always maintained and still do now, that I do not claim to have all of the answers to every question that arises as I go through this journey we call life. I have said, "I will Go On," and I sincerely mean it. I have never, ever considered abandoning my Faith, no matter what has come into my life. If Job of the Bible, Mother Teresa, and above all, Christ in the Garden, can go through times of loneliness, disillusionment, and feelings of abandonment, certainly we have to be honest with ourselves, that we too will encounter these times. That brings me to today's topic about which I chose to write.

It occurs to me today in a way that seems like a first. God has been with me through all of my life and I chose to follow Him at the age of 14 while attending a Billy Graham Crusade in Anaheim, California. It is something I have thought and re-thought—"Why would God allow this Parkinson's Plus to come into our lives if I have chosen to walk with Him and dedicated my life to His purposes?" I have confused this question with the original question. That question is—"Who do I believe He is and why do I choose to believe?" These matters are at times complex and we tend to make them so.

Today it seems as clear as that first moment I believed. Understanding everything is not required. Answering every question that we have about why we are here, why difficult circumstances are a part of the lives we live and what God makes of the way the world has gone in the last several decades, are great questions, but not the issue when it comes to determining our Faith.

It isn't just a matter of claiming that this human existence isn't valued and we should just believe for the sake of our afterlife and the eternity He promises. It isn't that simple. If this period of our eternity—the time He has given us with our families and friends on this wonderful earth—was to be overlooked, under appreciated and just considered a rehearsal for life in the hereafter, why would He have gone to the lengths of creating such beauty, order and promise?

Why would He provide the blessings and opportunities that He affords us, including me, one who has so much for which to be thankful? No, our human years do not dim as a result of choosing to walk with God in faith. If this life were to be taken for granted, why would our Christian truths be founded in the great value of the human life Jesus gave on the cross? This life was precious and to be highly valued by Christ Himself,

> *"Who being in very nature God, did not consider equality with God something to be grasped, but made Himself nothing, taking the very nature of a servant, being made in human likeness. And being found in appearance as a man, He humbled Himself, and became obedient to death– even death on a cross!"*
>
> *– Philippians 2:6-8, The Holy Bible, New International Version*

He went to the cross, not overlooking His 33 years as God in human form, but rather to demonstrate the amazing gift He was willing to give of His life on this earth.

Once I am able to see the distinction between these two issues—the gift of life on earth and the tremendous price he paid for our eternity—the clarity returns. I am able to give thanks to God for the value of my wonderful experience as a husband of the greatest wife and friend a guy has ever had. I see it as a privilege to be the father of three wonderful and talented sons and a gifted daughter-in-law. I recognize the treasures of close family and friends that have stood by me throughout my illness (you know who you are). I recount the blessings of doors God opened for me in my career as an educator, and I am able to give appreciation for the pleasure of singing the songs He has given me from the time of my high school years. Above all, I say "Thank you, God," for the grace He bestows on my life through the forgiveness of sins as a result of His amazing obedience on the cross. With these matters clear in my mind, I can begin to regain that child-like perspective.

It is too easy to confuse disillusionment over disease, hardship or struggle, with God's intentions for our lives. My wife and I have discussed this in great detail. We have come to the conclusion, and there are plenty of examples to find in the Bible, that God doesn't always promise to fix the human problems we encounter, including pain, hunger, disappointment, loss and depression. But if we ask Him, He will help us in the spiritual realm. Our spiritual issues do not go neglected. He said,

"And surely I am with you always, to the very end of the age."– Matthew 28:20, The Holy Bible, New International Version

This speaks to the constant presence of God in our lives, even through the greatest of trials.

Jesus went to the cross and was not rescued. He could have demanded this, but He chose to give up His human life, willingly. This speaks to the distinction between what God will allow us, by His grace, to experience in our human lives, and the promise of eternal acceptance by our loving Savior. This life on earth He has given us is a beautiful and rich source of fulfillment. As my wife explained, the essence of our faith is that the value God placed on our human lives is demonstrated in the greatness of the sacrifice Christ was asked to make on our behalf. He gives us an abundant life on earth, and in the afterlife as well.

I am thankful today that I have friends to talk through issues such as these, and I thank you for your patience.

More than anything, I want to let my wife know, her willingness to stand with me, physically, getting me through each struggle, and to have all of our long and deep conversations, really make a difference in my understanding. She has taught me so much!

Today feels like a new beginning, again. How about you?

A Poem: Posted on my Blog by an Anonymous Friend

I have heard you and I have felt you,
I can see you. You haven't disappeared, you haven't become less

Even though this earth is toiling against your body.
When your spirit swims the currents strong,
When the courage dims and when the anger moves from
ebb to tide...
Know that you have been faithful,
Know that you my child, my son, my victory,
You honor me and you have given me my due in worship.
Your life has brought and continues to bring me honor.
Carry on.
–speaking the Spirit to yours.
Posted by an Anonymous Friend

Some Things are Better Expressed in Music

"Through Your Eyes"
Words and Music
Dr. Daniel Brooks 2007

Sitting here wondering what to say
Sitting here wondering what to do
Knowing that my words, just won't be enough
To tell you, what you mean to me.

I've watched the world as it changes
Isn't really someplace I want to be
When the time arrives, it just won't be enough
To hold me, the way you've held on to me.

I'll follow you
You know the times we're going through
I could never see, the way you do for me
I want to see the world
Through your eyes.

Through your eyes, through your eyes
See the world through my disguise
I could never see, the way you do for me
I want to see the world
Through your eyes.

I've heard the wind blow through the trees
I've seen the soldiers on their knees
Every time I cry, and pray for their relief
That you will hold them
The way you've held on to me.

I'll follow you
You know the times we're going through
I could never see, the way you do for me
I want to see the world
Through your eyes.

Looking at the hatred
And the hunger
And the wars!
You've got to help me see,
My eyes are blinding me—
I want to see the world through your eyes.

This song was written to be recorded on my third CD, in progress at the time of this writing. It emerged out of the angst I feel
for so many reasons, but primarily a fresh view of life that comes
when you are faced with a neuro-degenerative disease. I have
strong feelings of loss, but also of a special kind of hope that I
will see life through a different set of lenses. I have seen things
that have changed me and I won't be returning to a view of the

world, or life itself, that I once held. We must grow, and as we do, we learn to leave things behind. There is a special freedom and renewal that comes with finally seeing things that have always been right in front of you, but they somehow evaded your awareness and attention.

Chapter Seven:

My Family and the Events that Shaped My Life

HAVE TOLD you the story of my illness: the things that led up to my first signs of Parkinson's Plus and the progression of symptoms that led to my diagnosis and treatment. What I haven't told you is "my story," or basically my family background and key events in my development, from childhood to adulthood.

I do not plan to tell you my story completely, as such an account about any one person's life would take an entire book. I would, however, like to give you a sense of the boy I was, and the family from which I came, as these details will add clarity to the account found in the rest of this book. If you have read the previous chapters, you know that I am a happily married Christian man, with three sons, a former career in public education and a very strong love for my past time, playing, singing and writing songs. These are the main aspects about which I would like to tell you. However, as I begin this biographical sketch, I do want to step back in time and explain my family roots.

ༀ

I was born in Long Beach, California at Saint Mary's Hospital on June 20, 1955. My first few years of life are the most difficult for me to recount, as I was more of an object of those years than a participant! Well, an object of great love, I am sure. I was born a week after my father completed his bachelor's degree at a small, private Christian college in Costa Mesa, known at the time as Southern California College. Today this school is called Vanguard University, and has blossomed into a liberal arts college, in addition to preparing ministers for work in churches and missions for the Assemblies of God.

After my birth, my parents, my older sister Teri Ann, and I moved temporarily to Azusa, California so that my father could attend graduate school to get his professional ministerial education. He was attending California Baptist College, which is the same school that later relocated to Riverside, the city of my eventual home.

My father, Ronald Charles Brooks, was born in LaJunta, Colorado, on October 3, 1929. He was born into a family that had both a strong entrepreneurial background, as well as some involvement in church leadership and ministry. His parents were Donald Charles Brooks and Enid Evelyn Wadlow. He grew up in and around Long Beach, including years in Wilmington, California. In those years all around the area you would look and see the giant, steel grasshopper-shaped oil pumps dipping their noses to the ground as they pumped oil to the surface. These were still active oil fields in my childhood and I had several opportunities to play around and near these odd looking structures, particularly on Signal Hill, where my cousin lived with his family in the early 1960's. It was with these oil derrick covered hills as a backdrop that my father grew up as an active and warm-hearted young man. Dad was an athletic fellow and excelled at football, boxing and contests of strength such as pull ups or high bar tricks.

By the age of nine, my father was playing the guitar, and by eleven, he added a horse of his own to complete the picture in his attempt to become a cowboy. My grandfather, Donald, eventually got into the gas station business and my father worked at my grandfather's various stations around Long Beach from his middle elementary school years, on. After high school my father enlisted in the Navy and was on an air craft carrier during the Korean War. He worked in the chapel on the ship assisting the chaplain by directing all of the protestant services, speaking, singing and playing for his fellow seamen. Dad's experience in my grandfather's Mobile gas stations paid off, when after my father was educated to be a minister, successfully completing a bachelor's degree, he chose instead to work in the automotive field as a skilled mechanic. My father's career in the automotive industry continued throughout the years my siblings and I were being raised. My father was a very good provider.

My father's mother, Enid, was a spiritual inspiration to all of the children in our family. She was a devout Pentecostal Christian, and shared her beliefs with each of us through books and letters she mailed. She prayed for me throughout my life, and I am grateful for her spiritual insights. Remarkably, she is living today and in early 2009, will celebrate her 100th birthday. Her smile, kind eyes and sense of humor are treasured by all.

Just short of my third birthday, my dad's father died suddenly, sending shockwaves through our family. It was a tough circumstance for my father, just 28 years old at the time. To this day, I have great sympathy and appreciation for my father, who withstood this loss despite its devastating impact. My mother, grandmother, and my father's two siblings were all impacted by this disappointing turn. I can recall seeing my father's grief and great disappointment.

My mother, Marguerite Ada Brooks, was born in 1932, in Los Angeles, California. She was the child of a father who was a certified public accountant, following a distinguished military career in the United States Army. Grandfather Eugene Moyers, who was born in 1891, served alongside Dwight Eisenhower in France during World War I. His knee was injured in battle and he walked with a cane throughout his life from that point on. Eugene married my grandmother, Maude Eva Barnhart, after meeting her in a Los Angeles music store, where they both were working at the time. My mother experienced frequent moves with her family around the United States, including Washington D.C. for a period of my mother's younger years. Several years were spent in Utah during World War II, and other years in San Diego. My mother still considers San Diego her other home town.

Marguerite grew up enjoying music, particularly. She enjoyed singing and eventually took voice in order to learn arias from various operas. She was an avid reader, and loved the public library where she would sign up for summer reading programs. She was excellent at sewing and school work, developing strong organizational skills. I inherited my administrative side from her, I am quite sure, and my father would agree. She took piano lessons as a girl, loved playing with friends and was a fan of the old radio drama programs that preceded the availability of television. As a high school student, she moved in with a family and served as a nanny and tutor for three children, a great responsibility for a teen girl.

My mother's father, Eugene, passed away when I was ten years old, and he was given a 21 gun salute. I remember receiving a shell from the military rifle's used cartridge when she returned home from the memorial. My mother, like my father, finished college, but did so after raising four children. We were all spread out over a period of 17 years, with the oldest being Teri Ann, born in 1953, the youngest Casey Andrew, born in 1970, and in the middle was my brother, Matthew Charles, who was born in

1962. My mother had her career development and education interrupted by the responsibilities of raising my siblings and me, as she focusing on homemaking and the training and nurture of my brothers, my sister and me.

Marguerite's mother, Maude, lived a full, active and self-sacrificing life, and passed away in 2001 at the age of 97 years. This was a great loss and I was honored to serve as officiate for the services and give the eulogy of her inspiring life. My brothers, Matthew and Casey, played and sang beautiful music to honor her memory. Maude was a Baptist and practiced regular Bible reading and prayer. She wrote insightful letters regularly to all of her family and thus inspired many. Grandmother Maude was in many ways the cornerstone and spiritual leader of her entire extended family.

My mother is still living in the same Lakewood home in which all of the Brooks children in our family grew up together. She has beautifully maintained the interior and exterior, and has done wonderful remodeling over the years. It is immaculate, though built in the early fifties. My parents bought that home used in 1958 for $15,000 dollars. It goes without saying that it has gone up in value many, many times more than its original price. It contained one bathroom and three bedrooms, crowded for a family of six, but it was a cozy and warm place in which to grow up. I generally shared a room with my brother, Matthew. The family room was an addition, with a step down and a big, used brick fireplace.

The builder of this inviting family room was our step-grandfather, Ralph Flory, who is one of my most beloved family members and heroes. Ralph was the second husband of my grandmother, Maude. He was the only grandfather I had the opportunity to get to know and the one with whom I spent the most time. Helping him build this room, with my small contributions, made my 11th year of life a time I will never forget.

My mother was still raising my younger brothers, Matthew and Casey, when she began to go to community college part time, and worked her way toward her associate in arts degree and then graduated from California State University, Long Beach with her bachelor of science in communicative disorders. These degrees were followed by her master of science in counseling, also from CSULB. She wasn't finished yet, and eventually completed her school psychologist's license and entered into a twenty-five year career in public schools as a psychologist. My mother did much to raise me, making sure I was focused on my education, ensuring that I had many sports and recreational experiences and carefully trained me to be a good citizen. She paid great attention to detail and her organizational skills influenced me, as I headed toward an eventual career as an administrator and leader.

My father was inspirational, giving me his penchant for performing music and impressing me with his evangelical training. He was one who believed in a Christian faith that would influence everything you would do, including each and every important decision, and that God's will for one's life was something that would unfold as you progressed toward manhood and chose your calling or profession. It was because of my father's love for his faith, that I made a decision to be an evangelical Christian and my earliest career goal became that of a professional minister.

Our sister, Teri, two years older than me, raised her family and then went to work in various capacities, including bank teller, automobile finance assistant, and retail store assistant manager. She has such a heart for people, and now works in a service capacity, in a medical clinic that treats cancer patients. My brothers are both excellent public schools teachers, each with many years of experience. Matthew, seven years younger than me, became an upper grades elementary teacher, serving in leadership within his union and was selected as a mentor teacher. Casey, born as I was about to turn 15, enjoys teaching the primary grades and is a bilingual teacher who can speak, read and write in Spanish. Teri sings beautifully. Matthew is an accomplished guitarist and singer, performing as an avocation with his band he founded and developed. Casey too has led his own country bands and plays guitar, along with several other instruments. He has enjoyed playing music within his church for many years. I am blessed to be related to such talented adults!

You can see that my siblings and I have chosen areas that are about serving the needs of other human beings. I am proud of each of my siblings and parents, for the care and concern they have shown for others. My Mom has recently retired but continues in the psychology field as a consultant and remains active in her love of travel. Dad still plays and sings as a guitarist in various assisted living and convalescent homes, as both an entertainer and minister.

∾

Lakewood was a community built right, with parks and fields every few miles and beautiful, well equipped schools. My home was down the street from Monroe Elementary School and a half mile from De Mille Junior High. Another mile down the road was Lakewood High School. My life was filled with consistency in that I eventually went to Monroe in first grade and would go through all of these schools without ever moving or having to adjust to a different environment. I say, eventually, because in my years of preschool and kindergarten, I went to Mark Twain, a school that provided extended day care for school age children. My mother was working during these years, and I went to the preschool and kindergarten for a full workday, until I reached the beginning of first grade, when my mother would stay home and I would return to my neighborhood to go to school at Monroe.

While in preschool and kindergarten at Mark Twain, I developed a great deal of inner strength. This was a public school program, and I remember well the numbers of children that would share the playground and eat the institutional cafeteria food together at a long table. I recall being required to take naps, and as a young boy, I had no purpose for sleeping at school. I remember the strict, physical discipline that was used when I wouldn't sleep with the mass group of children lying on mats. I had the top of my head plunked with an ink pen enough times to remember how it hurt and this gave me less confidence in the adults who were our caretakers. I was feisty enough to fight on the playground, as a three year old boy. This is where I learned to fight for myself for what I thought and what I wanted.

Kindergarten was a delightful experience of artistic expression and personal development. We painted with finger paints, crocheted yarn and made paper bag turkeys. I loved the art and the stories, in this very nurturing, developmental environment. I had some fearful moments when we were staying late after school, extending the day beyond the half-day kindergarten. We were being watched in a population age range that went from kindergarten to sixth grade, but I had my sister there to watch out for me. Teri was always watching out for me throughout our growing up years, and I know that her protection and affection for me has been a major influence over my life.

In the fall of 1961, a year before the birth of my brother Matthew, I enrolled in Monroe School and was placed in Ms. Conant's first grade class. I remember her response when, in the first five minutes of school that September, I read the names of colors on the front wall. Never mind the fact that the color words were printed on the paper flags made from the same color as the word printed on each one! Ms. Conant's compliment made me beam with pride and I began to develop well, particularly in English and Reading. My teacher indicated on my report card that, "Danny excels in writing and reading."

This community became a secure and happy world in which I felt very comfortable and in which I would flourish. The group I went to school with generally progressed through the grades with me, as our school size was booming in a burgeoning neighborhood filled with working class homeowners. A number of fellow students went through school in my class and eventually went with me all the way through high school. I feel very fortunate that our parents would work so hard to provide such a pleasant and secure community environment in which the four of us were brought up.

In these early years, we attended the local Presbyterian Church, which was within a half mile of our home. My mother had been raised in a Quaker Church, while my father was brought up Pentecostal. Initially, the Presbyterian Church wasn't ideal for either of my parents, but they had the ability to join forces and provide a church upbringing and education in a practical and close proximity to our home. This turned out to be a great decision, leading to my involvement as a high school student, in the youth group. For the most part, I had a positive experience in this church, although I remember being forced to sit outside the door for talking and goofing around during second grade church school class. I remember the feeling that I was frustrating the teacher and somehow continuing to do so until her breaking point was reached. I was not as interested in church school for a few years after that, but once I reached the fourth grade, I tended to want to go to church and I was likely to bring up the idea myself.

The neighborhood was filled with kids, and our street, six house lengths from the school, had children in each and every rooftop that would zigzag all over the front lawns of each other's homes and play long, sweat producing games of touch football in the street. What struck me about the neighborhood was that each family had a mother who was at home, most of the time. The fathers, taking a traditional role, were working, mostly in blue collar or skilled jobs. My father, from early in my elementary years, was not using his bachelor's degree in church ministry and Biblical studies, but instead chose to use his family given skills of auto repair. My father made a very good living as a mechanic working at various Chrysler dealerships in the 10 mile radius around our home. My father was one to work every day, with a single week of vacation taken every summer to drive to a cabin we would rent in the San Bernardino Mountains, so that we could swim and play at Lake Gregory. He never missed a day of work, unless he was severely injured or throwing up with the flu.

Every five to seven years, his dealership would sell to a new owner, or business would slow, which would result in his moving to a different dealership. With the exception of some of the earlier years in my childhood, my father was always able to find solid employment in the car business. I attribute this to his being a friendly person, gifted with people and possessing a natural sense of humor. I marvel at my father now when I realize the severity of his loss of his father when he was only 28 years old, and yet he maintained his cheerfulness and warm heart toward neighbors, customers and neighborhood children.

Often, I remember seeing my father standing in the front yard playing his guitar and singing for the children who would pack the porch steps, seated before their idol. This impressed me and I wanted to learn to do the same. By seven, he was teaching me chords and at eight years old, he was coaching me as I followed his chords and lyrics as his rhythm guitar player. The impact of this loving instruction would equip me for my life in ways that I cannot begin to measure in their worth and value.

I benefited a great deal from the wonderful opportunity to remain at Monroe Elementary School throughout my first through sixth grade years. I have memories of several highlights. One revolved around my school related experiences. Because I became a teacher and principal, I am inclined to mention school events in my history that involved the teachers that stand out in my mind. In second grade, I particularly enjoyed making butter in a jar with pure cream from a dairy. We shook it as it was passed around the classroom, and then it was spread on saltine crackers. We all enjoyed the wonderful flavor of freshly "churned" butter. This experience preceded our visit to an actual dairy, which were plentiful in the early sixties. By the late sixties, the dairies began to disappear in favor of the construction of the 605 (San Gabriel) Freeway, the development of Cerritos mall and the suburban homes that would eventually surround it.

This modern highway was built along the San Gabriel River, which still runs from the San Gabriel Mountains above Azusa, all the way to the ocean in Long Beach. My father and I actually rode our horses up on top of the unpaved road, with its fresh dirt that the earth movers had so expertly spread and smoothed into the shape that the freeway still has today. It was a great feeling of liberty to feel the wind in my face and the leather reigns in my hands, as I guided my mount along side my dad, while he road his favorite horse majestically toward the mountains to the north.

I was held after school in the second grade for talking in class, and when I walked outside to go home, I passed through a deserted playground. Along the way, I found a husky boy a couple of years older than me, swinging a belt over his head at a girl about my age. He was, from my standpoint, trying to whip her. All I know is that something inside me said to "stop this dangerous behavior," so I pursued him on foot and yanked the belt from his hand, shouting, "Leave her alone!" He resisted and as he glanced at me, he thought I looked like an easy mark. As he made an attempt to swing at me, I caught him first with a closed left fist and he quickly scurried off to his home, afraid of my potential prowess. It was then that fighting became a habit for me.

In third grade I remember being concerned about acceptance from friends and felt it was difficult to win the approval of the popular crowd. I was embarrassed by my teacher when she insisted that I turn my paper the same direction as the others in my class, though I was the lone left hander. I remember thinking she was ridiculing me, and I was ashamed for being different. I had to learn to write in long hand, in an over-the-top, hand curling manner because she slanted my writing paper to the left at the top, as she insisted that all the other third graders in my class were to do. I complied and became good at handwriting, but always wished throughout my years, including college and later as a teacher, that I could have been taught to write in a mirrored approach to my right handed peers, with my paper properly turned to the right at the top. I think this would have saved me from smearing all my papers and might have prevented me from having the huge hand cramps I experienced all the years I used a pencil or pen on any lengthy prose.

I was placed with Mrs. David for my fourth grade year, and she recognized some of my individual interests and abilities. She was the first to put me on a stage to play and sing for my fellow students. She also asked me to teach a female student to play the guitar, so that we could perform together. It was 1964, and the occasion was the annual fourth grade Thanksgiving program. I played a song or two with my first guitar student, Cynthia Weeks. We sang "I Ride an Old Paint" and "Home on the

Range" for the entire student body and I loved it! I was hooked on performing from that day on. Cynthia would later become the first to pass away after our class of 1973 graduated from high school. Looking back at Cynthia's fate, I was forever grateful that I had taken the time to teach her to play.

That same year, I was pummeled for the first time by an older student. I had a conflict the day before with a boy who picked up my half dollar when I was playing a game where you throw it from your elbow and catch it before it hits the ground. I had arranged to buy a St. Christopher necklace from a fellow student to give to a girl, and I was very aggressive with Cary when he picked it up. When he didn't give it right back at my request, I punched him squarely in the mouth, his previously chipped and pointed tooth cutting my left hand behind the middle knuckle. What I didn't know, was that this was going to get me into a fix I would have difficulty getting out of the next morning.

As I walked through the gate before school, I was approached by a much taller boy, who was in the sixth grade. He was apparently waiting for me in order to force me to fight another fourth grader I was better matched with than the boy I had the confrontation with the previous day. I was going to have no part of it, as he was taking me to fight the legendary Ronnie McQueen. Ronnie had the biggest biceps in the fourth grade and could perform miracles on the high bar! As my tall assailant, with a last name of Tyson, grabbed me, he sneered, "Come on. You are going to fight Ronnie." I pulled away in self defense, telling him, "No, I am not going!" When he attempted to grab me one more time, I swung at his face, hitting him hard in the jaw. Bad decision—or was it? This bully put me in a firm headlock under one arm, and then proceeded to punch me in the skull with his freehand, repeatedly, and I mean over and over! I just remember the pain and the feeling of being hit on the top of the head as though with a rock, and praying it would end. I was lucky in this second altercation to be exonerated, as I was in the first conflict I had experienced two years earlier.

Mrs. David taught me so much about the Japanese culture and I thoroughly enjoyed making wooden sandals, sewing a culturally authentic robe and sanding square dowels into chiseled chopsticks. We even carved replica California Missions out of Ivory Soap. The importance of these hands-on activities stayed with me throughout my years as a teacher, until I was eventually assigned as a principal at a school where I led the planning of a visual and performing arts magnet program. Twenty years later, I would coincidentally be at a Teacher's Association of Long Beach board meeting where I would have the pleasure of seeing Mrs. David honored at the end of her career as a successful and influential teacher. I hadn't seen her one time since the fourth grade, and there she was receiving an award at the end of her career! I took the opportunity to shake her hand and thank her for the things she had done in my life so many years before. The last I heard, she was living in the Palm Desert area of southern California.

My mother bought my first literature books that I could call my own in 1965, and two of the selections stand out. A Wrinkle in Time, by Madeleine L'Engle, and The Lion, the Witch and the Wardrobe, by C.S. Lewis, have become my favorite books throughout my life. The content of these books was very appealing to me and had an important role in my development. I became a science fiction and juvenile fantasy literature enthusiast. To this day, I have a passion for everything C.S. Lewis and M. L'Engle wrote throughout their lives. In addition, these juvenile fantasy books gave me a reason to want to become an elementary teacher, an idea that I developed as early as the age of 13. It is amazing how these books my mother decided to purchase for me made such a difference in my life spiritually, academically and professionally. I will forever be thankful for what she did in introducing me to fine literature that was to become the fabric that bound my heart to concepts of faith and a vision for dreams that could become reality.

I was a reader throughout the coming years, checking out books at school and avidly reading them on early Saturday mornings when I awoke and waited for the rest of my family to arise. I loved Matt Christopher books about sports and read with eagerness adventure stores about pirates and castaways. Robert Louis Stevenson's, <u>Kidnapped</u> was a memorable selection during these years.

Mrs. Cunningham, my fifth grade teacher, became my favorite teacher in elementary school. Young, smart and pretty, she encouraged me greatly and was willing to read, <u>A Wrinkle in Time</u> aloud for the class at my request. Years later, I was a young substitute teacher at another local elementary school and she walked into the office when I was picking up my classroom keys and written instructions for the day. I greeted her, and she remembered me, calling me, "Danny," which was the name I went by all through high school. I was thrilled to see her and in awe to be able to tell her I had become a teacher. She seemed quite pleased that I remembered her.

I disappointed Mrs. Cunningham one afternoon after it was reported to her that I had punched another student during recess. I saw a boy throw a ball at the head of a girl named Cheryl Bush, for whom I had developed a fancy. Seeing this attack, I ran over and punched him. Somehow, I was forgiven, because I was helping the female student who was struck by the ball intentionally. Another incident involving fighting at school and I had come out smelling like a rose.

It was at the age of 10 years that I awoke one morning to realize that my neck was very stiff and my head was nearly stuck to my left shoulder. I had a hard time lifting it and I could not turn my head. The pain was excruciating. My mother took me to an Osteopathic doctor, who did a maneuver much like a chiropractor would. He had me lay on the table and pulled my head away from my shoulders. Kind of scary for a young guy, but he was a great doctor that my mother trusted. When I returned to school, I had a strange neck brace on and I was very embarrassed by my appearance. The reaction I got stayed with me and gave me a sense of feeling odd and different from my peers. To this day, I wonder how much that early neck difficulty relates to other spinal problems and movement disorder issues I developed as an adult. I have thoughts about how much this neck stiffness and contorted posture I experienced as a boy was like the condition known as Dystonia, no matter how temporary it might have been at the time.

In the sixth grade I was able to become more popular, trading in my violin and "second chair" status in the school orchestra for an electric guitar I had received the previous Christmas. I joined a rock band with four other sixth grade boys. We played at parties and our song list consisted of selections by the Monkeys, the Animals and the Rolling Stones. My role was lead guitar and vocalist. We were known as the Knight Riders and once won a battle of the bands at the local parks and recreation clubhouse in our Lakewood neighborhood. Interestingly, the singer from the other band went on to be a part of the group, Kansas. He replaced Kansas' first lead singer. His brother, also in the band we battled that day, wrote songs that Kansas recorded. I was the other musician, between the two bands, that went on to pursue music in a serious way.

My sixth grade teacher, Mrs. Sprague, pulled me to the front to have a personal conference with me on the last day of school. She showed me my improved grade in English, which was a "B." I earned this by getting a "C" average for the first half of the year, and by getting nearly all "A's" in the second half. She said she expected great things from me in English and this was her evidence of what I could do. That conversation changed the course of my life, as I thought of myself as a language arts person from that day on, throughout my school career. I think this was a pivotal moment in my education and gave me the strong impression that I should communicate similar praise, when deserved, to my own students I would instruct years later.

During my late elementary years, my father introduced me to horseback riding. Our family rode horses along the San Gabriel River, and there were several riding stables where one could rent a horse and ride for an hour, at the price of a dollar or two. Soon after starting to ride with our father, our family then purchased a total of four horses, though we never had more than three at a time. My brother Matthew, who was between four and seven years old during this period, mastered riding as a young fellow. We kept our horses at Bob Buell's Stables, known as B and B. There were other stable businesses along the same river, including Spiller's and Broken Spur. I became serious enough about riding, and wearing cowboy boots and hats, and those symbols became a big part of my identity. Our family spent most of every weekend in this activity between the years 1965 and 1968. My mother and father would enjoy going on rides to lunch at the nearest Sizzler, which was an environment with a sawdust floor that sold primarily hamburgers and steaks; the salad bar and full menu of today is a complete departure from the original set up of these restaurants. Our parents literally tied their horses to the hitching post outside the door as they went inside to eat with their friends.

My sister, Teri, and I would ride with great interest. One year we entered a horse show, and we each competed in a contest—with my sister riding the barrel races and I chose the keyhole race. I have a second place ribbon for riding Blue Lady, a very fine horse that could run well and turn on a dime. Teri was very much a rider and enjoyed a barrel-chested quarter horse named Heidi, as did my father. Mom and Matthew rode Blue Lady most of the time, while I chose the so called plug horse, an older gelding named Pepe. I loved Pepe and was crushed when he turned up lame after a gallop with me through a trail along the river that was near construction. I was unaware for a few days that a nail entered the heart of his hoof. By the time my father realized what had happened, Pepe had turned up lame and was ill.

I watched with great sadness as he was hauled away in a trailer to be sold as a manufacturing resource. I will never forget looking in his brown eyes one last time as I climbed up the side of the trailer and peered into the window at what looked to me like a very sad face. "Good bye, old buddy. I love you and will miss you," I squeaked out through the square peep hole, as I fought back the tears. I learned to ride bareback and really grew in confidence and risk taking with that sweet old guy. I will miss him always.

My junior high years were filled with the pursuit of girls and learning the ropes of the academic world. It was during the eighth grade that I had the last fist fight of my life. It was a late afternoon, and I was at Monroe School, just down the street from home, working on my basketball skills. I was alone and taking shot after shot. A boy named Chuck Dolf, who was also 13 years old, walked up and I immediately sensed he was in a provocative mood. "Let me see the ball, Danny," he demanded. I said, "All right, but just for a minute. I need to get back to my practicing." Chuck took the ball and immediately threw it as far as he could in a northward direction, on the large, hard top playground on which we were standing. The school had virtually no grass on the fields. They were paved with black top made from tar and gravel. The ball bounced several times and eventually rolled for what seemed like blocks. It was literally over 100 yards, as the playground was a slight decline in that direction.

I was starting to boil and I directed Chuck to "Go get my ball!" He refused and I told him again, "Chuck, you had better get that ball!" Chuck continued to refuse and doubled his trouble by insisting that I fight him. He said, "Come on! Let's go!" and he began to kick the air, mimicking a kick toward my shins, while holding his two fists up and gesturing to come toward him. He persisted in asking and demanded, "Come on. Come on you (expletive)!" I was getting angry about the gall of this guy who would ask to see the ball just to throw it away, and then to have the nerve to demand a fight. "Chuck, I don't want to fight you. I don't want to hurt you. You go get my ball!" "Come on, Come on, let's go," he repeated. I warned him, "If we fight, you are going to be sorry." He waved his hands in front of himself as though boxing, and mimed the kicking motion in my direction.

Wham! I hit him with a left hook, something I was very familiar with since my father had brought me up boxing in the backyard. I was very sure of myself with my boxing skills and how to use my fists. Down went Chuck Dolf, and he was now on his back on the pavement. I didn't stop with that punch. This guy had driven me over the edge and I wanted to send a strong message. My anger raged and I leaned forward, swinging relentlessly for another minute or two, striking his face and forehead several more times.

"Okay, Okay! Stop!" Chuck cried. "Please stop! I'm sorry," he pleaded. I came back with, "Okay, Chuck. Get up. Get up and let that be a lesson to you. Get out of here and don't pull something like that again." I gave him a couple of half-hearted kicks to get him up and to reinforce that I wanted him out of my presence. He got up and began to run away. Now, you would think that would have taught him a lesson, but no, not this guy.

He got about 50 yards from me and stopped to signal with his middle finger to demonstrate his defiance—actually more an indication of his stupidity. He yelled, "I am going to tell my big brother to beat you up!" Well, he sure learned his lesson, don't you think?

Moments later, I retrieved my ball and went back to the court to begin to shoot and instantly realized I couldn't use my hand. The pain was excruciating and I looked down at my left and dominant hand, to see it begin swelling with blood before my eyes. I knew at once it was broken and was getting more and more painful each moment. It was worse in the morning and I got up knowing I had to confess to my mother. "Mom, I think I broke my hand," I started. She took one look at it and sympathetically asked, "What did you do?" I had to confess, "I got into a fight and hit Chuck several times in the head."

Mom told me to stay home from school and took me to see my Osteopathic doctor, who examined it and put on a cast, from my fingertips to my elbow. Now, I would have to write with my right hand for two months, something I had to learn to do and quickly. Also, my guitar playing became impossible, along with basketball, two activities I would hate to go without. My doctor told me, you have broken a bone in your hand and it has set slightly lower. He held up his hand and demonstrated what had happened, explaining why my first knuckle on my left hand was going to be permanently lower than the others. He told me, "Danny, you can never punch anyone again in this manner. If you do, I will have to put pins in your hand to set these bones together." I was so shocked to hear this prognosis and concerned that I would break these bones again, that I instantly determined never to fight again. I did not want to lose my guitar skills or be unable to swing a bat at a baseball. The way this part of my hand gripped a bat, it was the main location on my hand absorbing the force of the bat as it impacts the baseball thrown by a pitcher. I could not give up my dream of baseball and I certainly did not want to lose my ability to play my instrument. As it was, I had to wait eight weeks to get the cast off and then rehabilitate my hand in order to return to these serious interests.

I have thought of that fight as a blessing many times, as I was able to be the peacemaker in high school when tempers flared in basketball games that got too physical and almost resulted in fights. I became a leader and was captain of the basketball team, and usually the coolest head in the crowd stopping conflicts before they got out of hand. Before this broken bone and the lesson taught by my doctor, I was quick to take a swing at another boy for a small infraction. I did continue to box with my cousin or neighbor boys, but always using padded gloves that made the activity safe. I had a near brush with a fight in college when during a pickup basketball game on the Long Beach City College campus a big guy who was about my size got angry because of physical play and he punched me in the left cheekbone. I immediately realized, "If I hit him back, it could lead to an arrest and an expulsion from school." I simply looked at him and stated, "That's all right. It doesn't hurt that much." In reality, my left cheek did feel quite sore, but I didn't want this hot head to know. I wanted to put him on his back as I had done with Chuck Dolf five years earlier, but my good judgment prevailed and I stayed cool.

The next day, as basketball practice began, the same young man walked up and it was as though he had brought the red carpet under his arm to roll out just for me. He was polite and asked me to join his team for the day. He never again lost his cool and we became good acquaintances, never having another altercation. As a peaceful person, I have never had a reason to lay a hand on another man since the day I broke my hand on Chuck Dolf. In a strange way, by taking my ball that day, he had given me a gift for which I would always be thankful.

After I healed and returned to my activities, I continued to pursue sports enthusiastically, with five years of baseball, basketball and football behind me. If it was a weekend, I would be at the local park or baseball field, during each season of these three sports. I dreamed of the major leagues, growing up playing Little League baseball for seven straight seasons, from the age of 8 through 15. From the age of eight, I was on fall football, winter basketball and spring baseball teams, with never a missed season up through the ninth grade. Sports were my life, and I wanted so much to do well and make my parents proud. When I entered high school, I chose to play tackle football at Lakewood High School as a sophomore and also went out for the basketball team. In the summer prior to my first year of high school, I was playing senior league baseball, junior varsity basketball summer league, and participating in three-per-week football workouts in preparation for the fall football season. That was the summer I grew up and became a strong and resilient individual, giving up ALL of my free time, stressing my body to the maximum and growing in stamina and inner strength. I was a six-foot tall, 145-pound lean machine (Today I am six-foot-four and 250 pounds!).

Following my sophomore football and basketball seasons, I made the choice to stick with basketball, which, as I grew two more inches to reach six-foot-two and 165 pounds, became the obvious option for which I would be most suited. I fell in love with basketball, playing the center or power forward positions from that point on. I had a very successful season as an eleventh grader in high school, playing every game as the starting center on the Junior Varsity, leading the team in rebounds and scoring a few points in the post every game, as well. I was named captain and soon began to realize my potential for leadership, as I naturally found my niche in that role. There were a few boys that were better at shooting and they carried us in the scoring department, but I made my mark with rebounds, tough defense and managed to toss in a few shots in each game.

Meanwhile, I was an avid sports fan, falling in love with Major League Baseball, NBA Basketball and NFL Football, choosing to give my allegiance to the home team: the Dodgers, Angels, Lakers, and Rams. The Dodgers to this day remain my hobby and the Lakers, my passion. I remember the years of Jerry West and Wilt Chamberlain, as well as being a big fan of the Big Blue Wrecking Crew of the seventies, featuring Steve Garvey and Bill Russell, named here because they were my favorite players of the era. This is not to slight Piazza, Koufax, Magic or Kareem in any way shape or form. I am simply conveying the names that were the heart of my fascination with these two teams. I won't go into the Rams, mainly due to the reality that they were stolen from me and every other Rams fan in Southern California, when the late owner Georgia Frontiere moved them, without a thought for the feelings of the Rams faithful, to her own hometown of St. Louis in 1995. Shame on you, Georgia! You have left a big scar and a hole in my life that can't be filled.

My senior year I reached six-foot-three and 175 pounds, a good size in those times for a forward. The year soon became a disappointment as I made the varsity roster, but was forced to quit due to an injury to my left knee that was healing too slowly to realize my dream of a future in college basketball. Quitting, though painful, was the best thing that could have happened to my music plans. I began to perform for various events, such as sports banquets for several end of season awards activities, as well as playing for the annual Girl's League events. They liked my style of singing pop ballads and doing impressions of Elvis and the Bee Gees. It was in this senior year of high school that I began to see the future I had as a performer. My big opportunity came when the Long Beach Press Telegram sponsored a city wide talent contest that would choose one act from each large high school (six schools with 3,000 or more students, each) to join a troupe that would tour all of these schools, with each act doing a four minute spot.

I was generally the one solo act, playing guitar and singing. My act consisted of impressions of Ed Sullivan, Elvis, the Bee Gees and Bobby Sherman. I would end each impressions act with a trademark soft love song by Lobo, who had several top 40 hits in the early seventies. My act went over well at each of these large schools, where we would perform three assemblies, with each one containing a crowd of 1,000. This was a great experience for me and I realized that I loved the crowds, the lights and the adulation I was receiving. Eventually, I won third place in the city-wide contest, and our last performance was at the Long Beach Arena, the largest venue in the area at that time.

My crowning moment in my senior year was a concert I put on with a talented drummer by my side, as a fund raising event sponsored by the Ski Club. On a rainy January night in 1973, I drew 350 fans that paid 75 cents each to get in the Lakewood High School Auditorium, while the Rolling Stones played downtown seven miles away at the Long Beach Arena. I didn't receive a sports award as a basketball player, but in a poignant moment at the Senior Prom, I was given the trophy for "Most Talented Senior" for 1973 and the award was presented by the Varsity Basketball coach. I felt that I was soaring with a bright future ahead in music! As I graduated I had two clear goals: to get a college education for a career in church ministry, and to become a serious singer/guitarist. I felt that one or the other would become my lifelong career, and I was determined to be successful.

I was quite certain about church ministry as a career goal, and I would attribute that choice to my father's example and a youth minister I had at First Presbyterian Church of Lakewood. Reverend Jay Bartow brought a real difference to the high school youth program and it had a great impact on the lives of many young people. Through his mentoring, I grew in my faith and desire to lead. I eventually was leading worship with my guitar at the weekly home Bible studies he organized and was voted the president of the group in my senior year. His support and example made a great difference in my life, and a number of those whose lives he touched, are still professing the Christian faith today. The things Pastor Jay taught me about backpacking, trout fishing, social justice and above all else, the Christian life, are priceless treasures that have had a definitive impact on my life. I would need all of this and more as I finished high school and faced the real world.

$$\backsim$$

What I didn't anticipate, was the restlessness I would feel as I turned 18, a week after school ended. I was working at a busy car wash for $1.75 an hour, and determined that I could go out on my own on my birthday. I registered for the draft that morning, and by that evening, I had moved out of my family's home in Lakewood and into a downtown apartment in Long Beach. My life was about to change, drastically.

Being on my own brought challenges, financially and socially. Though I began college that fall of 1973, I was distracted by the freedom a young man enjoys, and inclined to socialize into the late night hours. I was playing in another band, this one with a couple of serious fellow musicians, a fine pianist/singer and my original drummer—both were outstanding. We began to play paid gigs and I developed further as a musician. Soon after, I became disillusioned with school enough to quit college and make an attempt at music full time. I was also tiring of the life I was living and my lack of focus. I worked odd jobs, struggling to eat on the hourly pay of a janitor at a private high school, cleaning late into the evening hours. As I did these jobs, I worked when I could, singing in restaurants and lounges, in the Long

Beach and Orange County area. Then, I had a Christian renewal experience that positively altered the course of my life.

Backing up for a moment, I was 14 years old when I went to a Billy Graham Crusade in 1969 and went forward to demonstrate publicly my decision to become a committed Christian. This decision was made with all sincerity and was the guiding force that I needed to get me through my early teen years. Though I had made a genuine decision to be a Christian, I lacked the maturity to remain solid in my commitment by the time I was living on my own, scraping to get by financially. Now, out of school, working hard for barely a living, I found myself sleeping on the floor, while splitting the rent for a studio apartment in a run down area of downtown. It was here that I began to sense God's call on my life. Across the street was a storefront church, similar to other non-denominational groups springing up during the Jesus Movement. This one was a somewhat immature, but sincere attempt to be a devout group of charismatic believers. I found the warm, welcoming environment both revolutionary and inviting. I began to attend with regularity and the things I had determined to believe earlier in my teen years came back to me in full force.

With the renewal of my Christian faith, I was inspired to begin writing songs that expressed my Christian beliefs. On December 31, 1973, I wrote the first of approximately 20 songs in a six month period. I sang these in churches, at youth meetings, camps and festivals. Some of these songs were good enough to stand the test of time, and many years later, found their way onto my first album released at the age of 40, in 1995. Over the many years that followed I continued to write and sing my own compositions, eventually writing well over 60 songs, but the period in my 19th year was my most focused time of writing, and remains so to this day. In recent years, after being diagnosed with Parkinson's Plus, I have written five new songs, the most productive period of song writing since these early years in my late teens. The impact of this life-changing disease has inspired me to write of the struggles it produces and the faith that I depend on, daily.

Returning to college in 1976, I worked my way through school as a teacher's aide, and although my goal was still church ministry, I began to realize that a career working in education was something I would have to seriously consider. I continued writing songs and performing as exclusively a Christian musician, and made a serious attempt with another band, called "Changing Heart." This group included another pair of outstanding musicians, a bassist/singer and a lead guitarist/banjo player, adding their talents to my songwriting, guitar work and vocals. Together we grew in our talent and knowledge of the Christian music field. This group lasted about two years and I have great memories of our southern California destinations at churches and Christian campgrounds where we sang and played for teens and young adults.

After a year in northern California as a youth pastor, I soon realized that my work as a teacher's aide in Long Beach had shown me my true career love—teaching. I returned in 1979 to Long Beach, where I resumed my education, with the goal of becoming a full time elementary school teacher. I completed my bachelor of arts degree in December 1980 and secured my first teaching position in early 1981, at Bret Harte Elementary School, in Long Beach. I taught the fourth, fifth and sixth grades and remained at Harte until June of 1986.

෴

In 1981, I began to attend a church with an active singles group ministry, where I would meet the love of my life, my wife of 27 years and the mother of my three fine sons. God provided me the partner and love that would fulfill all my dreams, and I know that Karrie was the woman I was meant to marry!

Our first date consisted of my attending an Easter musical at a large church in Anaheim, California. Karrie sang in the chorus providing the songs accompanying the musical theater production. After her performance, we went to dinner, followed by a walk near the ocean. I was hooked that very first night.

We were married on December 19, 1981, at a church in Costa Mesa, California. We settled in Long Beach, not far from the school where I taught fourth grade. Karrie and I had our priorities in order and we determined after our first son was born in 1983 that Karrie wanted to be home with Daniel, Jr., and I was very much in support of that idea. She made the decision to leave her position as a talented insurance claims examiner, with a bright future ahead. I have always appreciated the sacrifice of career enjoyment she made to spend better than the next two decades raising some wonderful young men. I, to this day, believe that this decision on Karrie's part benefited my sons, Daniel, Mark and Stephen, more than any other aspect of our lives. She made the difference and I am so proud of the courage and dedication she showed in giving these boys the best possible environment in which to learn and grow.

Daniel was three and Mark, born in 1985, was one year old, when I completed my master of arts degree at California State University, Long Beach. It was while I was in my last semester of this degree program, and working as a program facilitator/coordinator, that my first major medical difficulty struck. My spine had been injured during sophomore football practice in 1970, and it had troubled me all through the next sixteen years. It became worse when I moved heavy furniture and pianos in those early adult years. The wear and tear that comes from playing adult, city league basketball and softball, along with being an avid jogger, running in 10-K races into my late twenties, had taken its toll, also. Now, at the age of 30, I needed an operation to remove a seriously herniated disc in my lower back. The surgery was performed successfully, but the pain and difficulty that follow a back surgery of this magnitude, proved difficult from which to fully recover.

I moved from Bret Harte Elementary School to Clara Barton Elementary, which was also in North Long Beach. My role was program facilitator, which meant that I doubled as a vice principal. In this environment I had a chance to learn the principal position from a strong manager and leader, Mrs. Joan Taylor, who had an autocratic style, something I wasn't accustomed to in my young career. Joan had been my school counselor when I was in my elementary years at Monroe School. She was strong and affirming, and believed in me and my future. Before leaving her school at the end of the year, she walked me through the halls and encouraged me by saying, "I can see you with your own school one day. I can see you as a principal walking through the halls of your own school." Little did I know that this would be realized in the not too distant future.

During my year at Barton, the 1986-87 school year, I was responsible for preparing the entire school for a three day visit from state evaluators, a review known as Coordinated Compliance Review. There was much training and documentation to do in preparation and we did well when the review was completed and the report written. There were thirteen quality criteria that were the reference point in determining success or failure. Data and student work were compiled and collected, and I had 13 big boxes full of information that addressed the quality criteria being considered. The last thing I did at Barton was read the "report of findings" in front of the entire staff, parents, state officials and district dignitaries. At the conclusion of my seventh year as a teacher, with two being in the coordinator/facilitator role, I was in the mood to get back to my first love, classroom teaching. As I sought my next position, I was looking for a fifth or sixth grade classroom role in a developing area east of the Los Angeles basin, called Moreno Valley.

In August of 1987, we moved to Moreno Valley in order to take advantage of the affordable, new homes and with an obvious opportunity to progress in my career in a fast growing school district. Daniel was four and Mark two, and Karrie was expecting Stephen in December of that same year. I was in Moreno Valley for one year as a teacher before being selected to fill an assistant principal position. This was a challenging and time consuming position, but I soon saw how this type of work, as a school leader and manager, suited me as a person. I returned to post-graduate school for two years at night, driving 25 miles each way to get my second tier administrative credential. This certification was required to remain employed as a school administrator in the State of California. I remember the agony I felt when I would rush home from my assistant principal's office at Midland Elementary School in Moreno Valley. I would choke down a delicious meal Karrie had prepared and then drive away, leaving behind my three sons and Karrie, each with whom I desperately wanted to spend time. This took place two nights each week, for two years, in order to complete this additional certification.

Once I had a taste of administrative work, I was determined to become a principal of my own school. At 34 years old, after a second year as assistant principal, this time at Serrano Elementary School, I applied for and was selected for a position as a school principal, returning to Midland Elementary on the north side of Moreno Valley. From that beginning, in April of 1990, I remained a principal, with stints at four elementary schools and one middle school, for the next 13 years. I was given a number of awards, but the one I cherish most was the Principal of the Year I received, along with becoming a finalist for the county-wide honor, in 1994. This resulted from a staff wide effort to develop and implement Butterfield School of the Arts, a brand new magnet program that really was ground breaking. I am very proud of the teachers, staff, parents and students who worked with me to make this vision come to fruition. We created something at Butterfield that was truly unique in the school district as an option for students to apply for, and if selected, to attend.

The challenge was to create a program that would meet the needs of our own local attendance area, the neighborhood surrounding Butterfield, while creating a program that would attract students at large. Our surrounding community fed our school of over 900 students, and this coupled with 180 magnet students, gave us a challenging size of 1080. We were also asked to convert the school from a traditional year calendar to a 12-month, four track school, a program known as, "Year Round School." We accomplished all of this and garnered the attention of educators and parents throughout the school district.

During these years, my boys grew and we enjoyed the activities they chose and excelled at, such as baseball, basketball, soccer, and cub scouts. Karrie and I were always involved, with Karrie doing team mom duties and I serving as a manager, assistant coach or score keeper. These were very fulfilling, busy and happy years, providing us with many wonderful memories. Our sons were very fortunate to have the opportunity to attend one of the finest elementary schools in the county, Northridge School. We selected our second home in Moreno Valley knowing it would be a half block away from this beautiful, new school. It was one year from being completed when we moved into our house on Lombardy Lane that fall. A year later, in 1990, Daniel and Mark were in the original student body, with Mark starting kindergarten and Daniel second grade as Northridge Roadrunners.

Karrie was involved and on campus frequently, supporting the staff and students as a volunteer. I went to work happy, knowing my family was well taken care of and in a safe environment. A couple of years later, Stephen attended kindergarten there, before he and Mark moved over to Cloverdale School. It was during these years that Karrie returned to college and finished her degree at Riverside Community College. We were all so proud of her when we sat in the stadium to see her conferred with her diploma.

Along the way, I injured my back further in 1995 and needed a more involved and intrusive operation to remove discs from two areas of my spine. This operation was painful and involved a three-month recuperation period that threatened my future. If it were not for Karrie and the support of my sons, I might not have been able to get strong enough to return. I actually was able to continue on, and though I felt severe pain in the ensuing years, I continued to serve as a school principal. After five years at the helm of Butterfield, I was promoted to Principal of Landmark Middle School for the 1996–1997 school year. Noting much turmoil in Moreno Valley, Karrie and I decided we would sell our home and move our family to Riverside. We moved into a beautiful, new home on a quiet street in the Orangecrest area. We would stay in Orangecrest for 10 years, until Parkinson's Plus would dramatically change our plans, resulting in our moving back to Moreno Valley out of financial necessity.

After our family moved to Riverside, it was a natural decision for me to also move to a Riverside area school district, known as Alvord Unified, as the right place for me to continue my career. In my fourth principalship, I found my niche at a large year-round school in Corona City limits. I worked at Promenade for four rewarding years, and enjoyed a great staff, student body and parent community at this school. It was in my second year at Promenade that my back required additional surgery.

In 1999, the two levels of my back that had required disk removal in 1995 had weakened and developed scar tissue that was crowding my nerve roots. I was having difficulty walking and the nerve pain in my feet was severe. I went back for more surgery, and this time my orthopedic surgeon fused these two levels. This procedure would stabilize my spine enough for me to work another seven years as a school manager.

Meanwhile, Karrie developed a number of pastimes and pursuits of her own, in addition to managing the home, the finances and guiding our children. She attended a seven-year Bible study program for women that covered the entire Bible. After completing that course, she continued on with another weekly women's Bible study group that she still participates in today. Her artistic skills and love for crafts, led to the creation of some beautiful cards for friends, many craft-oriented decorations for our home and a number of memory book photo albums that chronicled our family over the many years. Each and every project, including painting and decorating our various homes, was done with creative precision that is unequaled. Her cooking for our entire family, and often the friends the boys brought home, was always delicious, amazingly organized and appetizingly prepared. She reads often, enjoys puzzles, is outstanding at handling finances, and writes beautifully expressive poems, when she has a bit of time. Her singing voice is featured on the album called, I Will Go On. It was a real joy to finally get to do a project together. You can hear us laughing with each other, as we worked until exhaustion in the studio.

By 2001, Daniel was in college and working in an after school program for at risk students. Mark was in high school and enjoying his many friends and playing drums in a band with his brother, Daniel. Stephen was racing bicycle motor-cross in Perris, California and attending middle school. Daniel received his Associate of Arts from Riverside Community College in 2002,

Mark received his high school diploma from King High School in 2003, and Stephen graduated successfully from King High in 2006.

I entered a doctoral program at La Sierra University in Riverside and received my Educational Doctorate (Ed.D.) in Education in 2003. Interestingly, Daniel's commencement to receive his bachelor's degree from California State University, San Bernardino, was at the same time that I was chosen to receive the Graduate Student of the Year for La Sierra University. The decision was never difficult—Daniel's graduation from college was my first priority, as I chose to skip the public recognition at the graduation ceremonies for La Sierra University. I understand that when they announced my award, the University President explained that I was prioritizing my role as a father rather than be present to receive top graduate student honors. It was exciting in June of 2003, as Daniel, Mark, Jenny, and I, all graduated from our respective schools. We had a wonderful celebration at our home with many close friends and family in attendance.

My long sought after career goal was a director of personnel position in the district office. I had become attached to the staff and students at my last school, Terrace Elementary in Alvord. The two years I spent at Terrace, a school with a decidedly lower socio-economic student population, were reminiscent of those I had spent many years before when my career started in Long Beach Unified School District. In 2003, I competed for and was appointed director of human resources in Beaumont Unified School District, after a grueling selection process. I was the director for two years, when the superintendent and board of education named me the assistant superintendent of personnel in the summer of 2005. By this time, I had been a teacher aide, classroom teacher, facilitator/coordinator, assistant principal, principal, director, and assistant superintendent over a thirty year period, in four school districts, which included: Long

Beach, Moreno Valley, Alvord, and Beaumont. I had enjoyed the students, parents, teachers, support staff and fellow administrators more than I could ever say. What a life—spent working with kids and leading adults!

In my last couple of years, I had to undergo a hernia operation and an appendectomy, on separate occasions. I know these two operations, performed under general anesthesia, added to the toll my three back surgeries had taken on my mind and body. In the summer of 2005, as I was promoted to assistant superintendent, I began to have my first pronounced head and hand tremors.

The boys were all progressing in their lives as young adults. Daniel had completed college and married Jenny in the previous year. He was starting his career as a school teacher. Mark had begun college two years before and had been on cross-country tours with his band, in which he was the drummer and background vocalist. Stephen was entering his senior year of high school and was developing into an accomplished artist.

⁓

By this time, I was becoming seriously concerned with the effect these tremors were having on me, and I began to notice the general lack of vitality I was developing. In addition, I was experiencing a depression that was deepening, gradually over time. We began to put the pieces together, and in hind sight, Karrie remembers noticing my lack of energy and constant falling asleep after work each day. The weekends brought more sleep and I walked slowly when out for exercise with my wife. I had balance difficulties and would sway in place if I closed my eyes while standing to pray with Karrie before leaving for work each day.

Later, in the fall of 2005, my neurological issues began to affect my walking gait, caused difficulties with effective speaking and led us to pursue a serious medical course to find answers as to why these problems were besetting me. I didn't get to finish my year as an assistant superintendent, becoming permanently disabled by February of 2006. Through the years leading up to my disability retirement, and along the way, I continued to hold to my Christian faith, with Karrie and I raising our family in a church environment, with consistency.

I was able to keep on singing and playing my music, hitting the coffee houses and church services over the years, to keep a small part of the dream alive. I did record another CD in 2006, entitled, "I Will Go On," focusing on the positive forward movement I would attempt to make, in spite of my eventual diagnosis of Parkinson's Plus. At the time of this writing, CD number three is in progress.

My difficulties with balance, an early progression of walking gait difficulty, speech troubles, eye movement dysfunction, a change in the coordination of my extremities, and mild cognitive changes that became noticeable, brought my neurologist to the Parkinson's Plus diagnosis. Faith, the priority of family, hard work, annual camping trips, enjoyment of music, love for sports, caring for beloved pets, and a simple, modest existence have remained the focal points of my life. I brought those things with me into this era of my life, life after PD Plus. I believe that since this disease has been part of my life for a number of years prior to my noticing the increasing symptoms, it is an important aspect of who I am. It always has been, irregardless of when I became aware of it, and it is not something that I reject, in that sense. It is part of the package of who I am as a total person.

I go on in life, with the neuro-degenerative disease, the desire to live my life to the fullest, the intention to walk with God, the will to enjoy my wonderful family and my deep appreciation for the beautiful world God has given us. My sons are doing well in life, with all three being musicians, each one in good health and all three possessing strong character and genuine concern for other people. The oldest is now a teacher in his fourth year, carrying on the tradition of educating the youth of today. Daniel's wife, Jenny, is also an accomplished teacher. Daniel and Jenny live in a nearby city in their own home, and take time to travel to a number of exciting destinations. Stephen was born at the time that we moved to Moreno Valley, making me a proud father of three sons, in 1987. He is now 21, a surprising reminder of the way the sands of time slip from our grasp. He is studying art in college, working at a sporting goods store, and enjoying his outdoor, wilderness-oriented activities. Our middle son, Mark, born in the midst of the years I was working on my master's degree, became an accomplished musician, recording a double album with his band and helping to produce my 2006 album, "I Will Go On." He is working with me now to complete the current project, and continues to go to college. Mark works nearly full time at March Air Base.

Karrie is still my best friend and lifelong partner. We are beginning our 28th year of our happy marriage. I am grateful to have had the very best wife a man has ever had, and, in my mind, her beauty is still unparalleled. She is an unselfish caregiver, and provides me with assistance, companionship, encouragement, and a shoulder to lean on. She transports me everywhere I need to go and makes sure I take my many required medications, without which I could not function.

Life is good. I have no way of knowing how much the spinal operations, other surgeries, and still the stress and strain of a very challenging career, played in the development of this disease, Parkinson's Plus. I just know that it all somehow factors in, to one degree or another. I will probably never know the cause of my illness. I am not asking to change it, but only that I may learn from the challenges, and, to as much a degree as is possible, grow through it. This will give me the best possible chance to beat the odds. Getting over hurdles is something I have been familiar with throughout my life, and I expect to continue overcoming for many, many more years ahead.

"I can do everything through Him who gives me strength."– *Philippians 4:13 – The Holy Bible, New International Version*

References

The following is a list of books that contributed to my knowledge and you may find helpful in facing a Parkinsonian disease.

Christensen, J. H. (2005). *The First Year – Parkinson's Disease: An Essential Guide for the Newly Diagnosed.* New York, N.Y: Marlowe and Company.

Church, M. J., & Garie, G. (2007). *Living Well with Parkinson's Disease.* New York, N.Y: HarperCollins.

Fox, M. J. (2002). *Lucky Man: A Memoir.* New York, N.Y: Hyperion.

Guten, G. N., Horne, J., & Tagliati, M. (2007). *Parkinson's Disease for Dummies.* Hoboken, N.J: Wiley.

Jahanshahi, M., & Marsden, C. D. (2000). *Parkinson's Disease: A Self-Help Guide.* New York, N.Y: Demos Medical Publishing.

Kondracke, M. (2001). *Saving Milly: Love, Politics, and Parkinson's Disease.* New York, N.Y: Ballantine.

Lang, A. E., Shulman, L. M., & Weiner, W. J. (2007). *Parkinson's Disease: A Complete Guild for Patients & Families (Second Edition).* Baltimore, Maryland: The John Hopkins University Press.

Lieberman, A. & McCall, M. (2003). *100 Questions & Answers about Parkinson Disease.* Sudbury, MA: Jones and Bartlett Publishers.

Lieberman, A. (2002). *Shaking Up Parkinson Disease: Fighting Like a Tiger, Thinking Like a Fox.* Sudbury, MA: Jones and Bartlett Publishers.

Marjama-Lyons, J. & Shomon, M. J. (2003). *What Your Doctor May Not Tell You About: Parkinson's Disease.* New York, N.Y: Time Warner Books.

Quigley, S. & Shroyer, M. (1996). *The Little Book of Courage: A Three-Step Process to Overcoming Fear and Anxiety.* Berkeley, CA: Conari Press.

Sacks, O. (1990). *Awakenings.* New York, N.Y: HarperCollins.

Disclaimer

I am not a medical doctor. This book was not written or approved by any doctor, neurologist, or licensed health care professional. The content and information contained in these pages were written by me, based on informal, non-quantitative research and personal experience as a neurological patient. Please consult with a licensed/registered physician to confirm the accuracy of what you read on these pages.
– Daniel Ryan Brooks, Doctor of Education

Made in the USA
San Bernardino, CA
22 September 2013